Insider's Pre-Med Guidebook: Advice from admissions faculty at America's top medical schools

ISBN: 9798720597818

Typesetting & Interior Book Design by Anamaria Stefan

SECOND EDITION

INSIDER'S
PRE·MED
GUIDEBOOK

Advice from
admissions faculty at America's
top medical schools

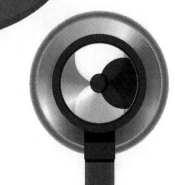

BYRON LEE, MD
ANDREW KO, MD
MATTHEW PETERS, MD
and SAMANTHA AN

Dedications

Dr. Byron Lee: To my amazing wife Tracy, our precious boys Isaiah, Aaron, Nathaniel, and Asher, and my parents Steven and Kammie who taught me to dream big.

Dr. Andrew Ko: To my dear wife and best friend Christine, our beautiful kids Naomi and Elliott, and my loving parents, Hsien and Jane, without whom I would not be where I am today.

Dr. Matthew Peters: To my parents, Mark and Su, for giving me the freedom to dream and the ability to achieve.

Samantha An: To my parents, Joni and Sam, and my brothers, Nick and Griffin, who are my unwavering support system.

Contents

Index of Info-Boxes

Chapter I

Is Medicine
Right for Me?

So, you want to be a doctor—or, at least, you think you do. Every year, hundreds of thousands of students pursue pre-medical studies at four-year universities across the United States and the world, and they, too, want to become physicians for a myriad of reasons. Many will find their reasons to be mature and well-reasoned. These students will find the motivation and strength to succeed as pre-med students, medical students, and physicians, and they will live happy and productive lives. Others will pursue medicine for reasons that are immature, underdeveloped, or untested. For these students, there are two major possibilities: they will struggle through their pre-medical studies and drop out, or they will end up dissatisfied with their life-long careers as doctors.

Before you pursue medicine as a career, you must be sure medicine is a good fit for you. If your motivations are poor or false, you will not have the drive to succeed during the long and difficult road ahead. You will lose time, money, and the opportunity to pursue whatever your passion truly is. If your motivations are genuine and well-developed, you will find this path to be easier and infinitely more rewarding. Not only that, but your passion will shine through the activities you pursue. Medicine is a pursuit that is simply too long, too difficult, too costly, and too important to pursue for the wrong reasons.

One of the most common questions during the medical school interview is "Why medicine?" An applicant's response to this question can make or break their performance on the interview, and, concomitantly, their entire application. As medical school interviewers, we have heard many different answers to this question. We have assembled some of the reasons we have seen for pursuing medicine. As you read through them, we hope you will notice a pattern: that the best reasons are formed through sustained medical experiences, while the worst reasons lack relevant insight.

Bad reasons

We often meet applicants who look absolutely amazing on paper. They appear to excel in every respect. Their grades, test scores, and extracurricular activities are excellent, and their life stories seem compelling. Their letters of recommendation drip with every superlative imaginable. They come from a great school and managed a rigorous course load. But when we interview some of these superstars and ask them a simple question—"Why medicine?"—they struggle to give a thoughtful and persuasive response. Despite their strong record, we often reject these otherwise stellar candidates. Here are some of the poor reasons that so often hamstring an applicant's chances of acceptance, and why. These reasons are occasionally explicitly stated by the applicant, but more often inferred by the admissions committee interviewer.

Reason 1: My parents have always wanted me to.

As an adult, you should be able to make your own decisions for your life. While you may have individual and cultural beliefs that place a high value on family desires, we nonetheless feel that medicine should ultimately be your decision—and nobody else's. When you are working 80 difficult hours a week during your residency, will it be your mother working that shift, or you?

Reason 2: My parents are physicians, and I want to follow in their footsteps.

Many pre-medical students come from homes where one or both parents are physicians. While growing up in a household of physicians may give you exposure to the field, it alone is not a sufficient reason to go into medicine. We are often wary of applicants who are the children of physicians because many have failed to explore other career possibilities. On occasion, they resign themselves to pursuing medicine out of convenience. You must be able to demonstrate that you want to be a physician because there are unique elements of the career that you particularly enjoy.

Reason 3: I want to make a lot of money.

According to the US Department of Labor, the annualmedian pay for physicians and surgeons was greater than or equal to $208,000 in 2019.[1] While these numbers may look particularly lucrative, physicians take home much less than these figures reflect.

Unlike many Americans who enter the workforce and begin to earn money at a young age, the average physician begins practicing medicine at a much later age. Before a physician can earn a large salary, she must spend her 20s earning a bachelor's degree and attending medical school. Those who graduated from college in 2020 paid an average of $141,825 for college tuition, fees, room, and board (in 2019 dollars).[2] Those who graduated in 2020 and attended an in-state public medical school paid a calculated median of $256,000. For private medical schools, the median cost increased to $338,000.[3] After medical school follows 3 to 8 years of residency, with average annual salaries of only around $57,000 in 2019, despite commonly working 70 to 80 hours per week.[4] In short, the loss of potential earnings, the cost of education, and the meager residency pay offset much of what physicians earn later in their career.

Even when one finally becomes a full-fledged, high-wage (and middle-aged) physician, taxes, malpractice insurance, and debt repayment take a significant chunk out of a physician's earnings. According to The Houston Chronicle, the average physician spends ten cents on malpractice insurance for every dollar you pay for healthcare, with some specialists paying considerably more just to stay afloat. Some obstetricians/gynecologists in certain areas of New York, for example, paid annual malpractice insurance premiums as high as $214,999 in 2017.[5] Medical school tuition debt can chip away at earnings for most of a physician's remaining life. A physician with $200,000 in federal direct loans might pay $1,600 every month for 20 years, with an interest of $221,000 ballooning the total repayment to $421,000, according to a 2019 AAMC report.[6] Lastly, the high annual physician wage obscures the fact that physicians work far more hours per year than the average worker, leading to a much lower hourly wage. According to a 2018 report by The Physicians Foundation, the average physician worked 51.4 hours per week, with many working significantly more.[7]

These figures indicate that a physician lives a relatively comfortable life—but hardly one that is extraordinarily lavish.

Reason 4: I want power and prestige.

In a 2016 nationwide survey, Americans ranked doctors as the most prestigious profession (with actors, stockbrokers, and politicians near the bottom).[8] Doctors and nurses both topped the list in a 2019 survey of America's most trusted professions.[9] With the white coat comes an undeniable sense of authority and trust. Why else do you see so many physicians endorsing products in commercial advertisements? Physician-themed TV dramas still remain a nightly staple of prime-time lineups, and parents hope their child will marry a physician, or so the stereotype still goes. There is also the allure of the power and responsibility a doctor wields—that another person's life is in your hands, and your decisions can decide whether someone lives or dies.

With physicians in the limelight of the public's psyche, it may be tempting to become a physician for the perceived social benefits that come with the white coat, stethoscope, and M.D. title after your name. But the truth is, in our experience, this reason is not powerful enough to motivate you during the tribulations you will regularly endure as a practicing physician. As a doctor, you will often feel frustrated and powerless when patients disregard your instructions, a treatment plan fails, or your ability to practice medicine is hampered by miles of bureaucratic red tape and a towering pile of paperwork to complete.

Reason 5: I want a job that is stable and always in demand.

According to the US Department of Labor, employment of doctors is anticipated to grow 7% from 2018 to 2028, which is faster than average for all occupations.[10] This growth in supply may not be able to keep up with the growing demand for doctors, especially as the populous baby boomer generation grows older and requires much more care.

While it is true that being a physician will become more of an asset, we hardly think the job security and market demand are good enough reasons to pursue the profession. For one, the job is not as cushy as it may seem. As doctors, we have missed important family obligations, events, and holidays because of the great and unpredictable expectations placed on those in our profession. Moreover, while the job is always in demand, employment is hardly guaranteed. While uncommon, physicians can lose their license to practice profession- ally when they perform egregiously. In 2003 to 2009, for example, 1 in 57 doctors lost their license in Illinois, compared to 1 out of 97 for lawyers and a similar figure for public school teachers.[11]

Most importantly, we would hope you choose to be- come a doctor for a reason that is more heartfelt and motivating than the cold pragmatism of job security. Many professions offer great job security—like teach- ers, nurses, and accountants—so why not pursue those jobs?

Questionable reasons

Some reasons to become a doctor are fairly poor. Other reasons are spot on. There are also some reasons that fall elsewhere along this spectrum, being neither completely good nor bad.

These questionable reasons have some elements that may be suspect, but they may also have some merits.

Reason 6: I can't imagine what else I would do. I've tried other things but did not like them.

If you interned at a law firm, a consulting firm, and a newspaper, and found you didn't like any of them, it doesn't necessarily follow that you must like medicine because you've exhausted other options. It is good to ensure that other potential fields are not for you—especially if you suspect you might like them—before entering medicine, but you must also be certain that medicine itself is right for you.

You may discover aspects of certain jobs that overlap with being a physician, and if you like those aspects, that may be an encouraging sign that you will also enjoy the practice of medicine. For example, if you enjoyed interviewing others for your news reporter job at your high school newspaper, it may mean you enjoy talking to patients and diagnosing their self-reported problems. Conversely, if you disliked your job as a waiter because you were "always on your feet talking to strangers," that may be a sign you will dislike most medical specialties, which require you to socialize and be on the go for most of the day.

That being said, none of these experiences can sufficiently gauge whether or not medicine is right for you. The only way to know for sure is to have clinical experiences. For example, if you enjoyed interviewing as a reporter, then you need to shadow a physician to see if patient interviewing is similar enough to what you liked about interviewing people for a news story.

Be aware that a doctor's day-to-day life can vary greatly, depending on their specialty. So, if you disliked one shadowing experience, do not assume you will dislike the entire profession. For example, if you disliked the frenetic pace of an emergency department physician, then follow a pathologist as he shows you his quiet, sedentary yet cerebral workday. You might like that better—or vice versa.

Reason 7: I got appendicitis when I was 14, and I admired how my surgeon treated me. Ever since my surgery, I've wanted to be just like her.

Learning first-hand what it's like to be a patient with a serious medical problem can be a powerful experience. The pain, fear, and uncertainty can give you a better understanding of what it is like to be a patient. You may develop a greater sense of empathy toward patients, and you can appreciate the human element that under lies the practice of medicine.

At the same time, many applicants with this kind of motivation often do not realize that a patient's experiences do not reflect a physician's. To evaluate whether you want to become a doctor, you have to approach it from the physician's perspective—after all, it is the doctor's shoes you will be filling, not the patient's. This kind of perspective can be gained through sustained, long-term shadowing and volunteering at your local care facilities, such as hospitals, clinics, and private practices.

Reason 8: I want to help others.

It's obvious that a physician's job is to help others. Healing is at the core of the profession. The problem is there are countless jobs that "help others." Lawyers help settle costly disputes, teachers help students learn, and nurses heal patients—just like physicians.

> **Box 1: An example of the right reasons**
>
> G.L. currently attends a top medical school in New England. As a teenager, she loved to paint and sculpt in her spare time. She was always good at science but never thought of it as a career. She was 19 when she became an aunt and her nephew was born with a cleft lip, which is a physical deformity right above the upper lip. As she learned more about the condition and the procedure to repair it, she began to see reconstructive surgery as an art form requiring a sense of aesthetics, dexterity, and manual skill, much like her passion for sculpting. She decided to shadow a plastic surgeon and volunteer at the hospital's children's wing. These experiences confirmed her interest in plastic surgery and medicine. She noticed that the patients she saw from socioeconomically disadvantaged backgrounds were more likely to require additional operations. While taking pre-med classes, she did epidemiological research on this hunch. G.L. applied to a dual-degree MD/MPH (Masters in Public Health) program to further her pre-medical interests in both surgery and epidemiology.

So why not become, say, a nurse? You must figure out what it is especially about physicians—to the exclusion of other professions—that you find unique and compelling. At the end of this chapter is a list of related fields you should rule out before deciding to become a doctor.

Good reasons

With all these wrong reasons, what, exactly, are the right ones? The common thread throughout all the poor reasons is a lack of thoughtfulness, focus, and experience. The best reasons to become a physician are grounded by a history of experiences that allow a pre-medical student to explore the practice of medicine. The most successful applicants to medical school pursue a depth and breadth of experiences that demonstrate a thorough, thoughtful, and unique exploration of medicine within a coherent narrative. Many pre-meds who pursue clinical experiences discover they want to enter medicine for the following reasons:

Reason 9: Physicians establish meaningful, long-term relationships with their patients.

Physicians average 1,800-2000 patients in their record books at any given time.[12] This figure hints at the vast and diverse pool of people a physician sees throughout his or her lifetime. As a doctor, patients will walk through your doors with a diversity of physical conditions, ages, languages, ethnicities, cultures, religions, beliefs, lifestyles, socioeconomic status, occupations, educational attainment, and more. This may range from an 82-year old Nepalese Buddhist monk who has hypertension (perhaps due to his secret predilection for American cheeseburgers) to a 28-year-old folk guitarist who develops a disease of the arteries due to his smoking habit.

As physicians, we have found that every patient has

a unique story to share, and each patient represents an opportunity to build an enduring and productive relationship. There is a special joy that comes from learning a patient's life history, keeping track of their successes and failures throughout their life, and seeing positive developments unfold due to your advice and treatment. Perhaps that 28-year-old folk guitarist will take your advice, stop smoking, improve his condition, get married, produce a hit album at age 46, and establish a cult following in Japan—or maybe he will ignore your advice, his limb will be amputated, he will take night classes, and work a 9 to 5 desk job in human resources. Who knows? As a physician, you get to find out what happens as you work with patients and establish longitudinal relationships with them—and that can be both exciting and rewarding.

Reason 10: Doctors are life-long learners, researchers, and educators.

Twenty years ago, a surgeon would leave a foot-long scar after removing a kidney. By 2007, a new technique was developed that allowed surgeons to remove the organ via a tiny incision in the patient's navel. This new procedure reduces hemorrhaging, minimizes post-operative scarring, lessens pain, and allows patients to be discharged from the hospital sooner. As a physician, you will be practicing for decades to come, and you will oversee new breakthroughs that produce better health outcomes.

You can also perform laboratory or clinical research that pushes the boundaries of what is known or translates what we discover into treatments we can actually use. Many physicians have made discoveries after pursuing questions that confronted them when they tried—and failed—to cure difficult cases. A famous example is Edward Jenner, an English country doctor who performed the first vaccination against smallpox after discovering that inoculation with cowpox conferred immunity. He based his theory on the observation that his patients who worked with cattle and had been exposed to cowpox never contracted smallpox, even after an epidemic had ravaged the community. He concluded that his patients' exposure to cowpox had unintentionally immunized them to smallpox.[13] As a doctor, you will constantly be learning, teaching, and perhaps even adding to the ever-progressing body of medical knowledge.

Reason 11: You can help others in a way that only a physician can.

Health is so important, and restoring it is one of the most impactful—and thus rewarding—ways you can help another person. As a physician, you get to restore health in a manner that is more executive than other health-related professions. Physicians are responsible for diagnosing illnesses, prescribing medications, and devising treatment plan. These responsibilities require a great deal of critical thinking, scientific reasoning, creativity, and leadership. To think, reason, and lead effectively, you must master your knowledge of medicine, maintain your professionalism, and keep your analytical skills in excellent shape.

Reason 12: Physicians have more autonomy, independence, and variety of practice than other health professionals.

Compared to most other health professionals, physicians have more freedom to tailor their career around their specific interests. Graduating with an M.D. degree opens one up to a wide variety of job possibilities, many of which are far removed from the hospital and clinic but are nonetheless medically relevant. Doctors increasingly earn dual degrees and pursue other fields, often as a way to fuse their passion for medicine with another related interest in a synergistic way. If you have interests in addition to medicine, we encourage you to pursue a career that incorporates both medicine and your other interests. However, do *not* pursue an alternative career if you have misgivings about medicine and feel an alternative career is a way to "compensate."

Career fields that incorporate medicine

- Academic research and teaching
- Alternative and complementary medicine
- Aviation medicine
- Business consulting
- Crowd medicine (festivals and public events)
- Executive recruiting (hiring and placing other physicians)
- Expedition medicine
- Forensic medical examination
- Healthcare administration
- Maritime and diving medicine
- Market research and finance
- Medical journalism, communications, and writing
- Medical law
- Medical photography
- Medical sales representatives
- Military medicine
- Pharmaceutical medicine
- Politics
- Prison healthcare
- Private and industry research
- Public and international health
- Space medicine
- Sports and exercise medicine

Related fields to rule out

While some careers may complement a medical degree, other careers offer similar duties, responsibilities, and experiences as that of a practicing physician. You should be certain you want to be a doctor rather than these comparable career positions:

- **Nurse practitioner**
- **Physician's assistant**
- **Dentist**
- **Podiatrist**
- **Pharmacist**
- **Optometrist**
- **Nurse specialist**
- **Physical therapist**
- **Chiropractor**

Summary

Before applying to medical school, make sure you have a good reason for why you want to become a doctor. Having good reasons will not only help you during your med school interviews; it will also assure you are more likely to be happy and fulfilled as a physician.

- Good reasons to be a physician tend to be grounded in personal clinical experiences that give you an understanding of what it is like to be a doctor. If you know and like what a physician does, you tend to have more mature, informed, and sophisticated reasons why you want to become a physician.

- There are other career fields that are similar to being a physician, and you may want to consider if those professions are more appealing to you.

- The field of medicine is quite diverse, and a medical degree can be a pathway to a number of jobs that may appeal to your particular beliefs, values, and interests (e.g., aviation medicine, forensic science, and military medicine). Consider whether a particular kind of medicine appeals to you.

---

[1] https://www.bls.gov/ooh/healthcare/physicians-and-surgeons.htm#tab-1

[2] https://research.collegeboard.org/trends/college-pricing/figures-tables/average-published-charges-sector-over-time

[3] https://www.usnews.com/education/best-graduate-schools/the-short-list-grad-school/articles/most-expensive-private-medical-schools#:~:text=Paying%20for%20four%20years%20of,for%20the%20class%20of%202020.

[4] https://www.aamc.org/system/files/2019-11/Survey%20of%20Resident%20Fellow%20Stipends%20and%20Benefits%20Report%20 2019-2020.pdf

[5] https://www.ama-assn.org/press-center/press-releases/ama-studies-show-continued-cost-burden-medical-liability-system

[6] https://store.aamc.org/downloadable/download/sample/sample_id/296/

[7] https://physiciansfoundation.org/wp-content/uploads/2018/09/physicians-survey-results-final-2018.pdf

[8] https://www.forbes.com/sites/niallmccarthy/2016/03/31/americas-most-prestigious-professions-in-2016-infographic/#249637541926

[9] https://www.forbes.com/sites/niallmccarthy/2019/01/11/americas-most-least-trusted-professions-infographic/#1dc00a27e94e

[10] http://www.bls.gov/ooh/healthcare/physicians-and-surgeons.htm

[11] http://www.huffingtonpost.com/leonie-haimson/factchecking-waiting-for-_b_802900.html

[12] https://www.physicianleaders.org/news/how-many-patients-can-primary-care-physician-treat

[13] http://www.ncbi.nlm.nih.gov/pmc/articles/PMC1200696/

Chapter II

How to be Pre-Med

Y ou think medicine is right for *you*, but are you right for *us*? Across the nation, medical schools will be asking themselves that exact question when thousands of students apply to their school to compete for the desperately few seats that are available to fill. With acceptance rates ranging from 2 to 7 percent, medical schools can afford to be extremely selective when they decide whom to admit and whom to reject. Knowing their fate is in someone else's hands, and perhaps lacking confidence about whether they have sterling enough credentials to impress, many applicants may end up psyching themselves out or compromising their integrity. How does a candidate remain true to oneself when it seems like so many around them may be trying to "play the game" to their best advantage? How does one put their best foot forward while maintaining integrity throughout the entire process?

It's easy to reel off the components of a medical school application that are taken into consideration in the admissions process, such as grades, MCAT scores, volunteer work, research experiences, personal story and background. Each of these measures and predicts an applicant's aptitude for the things that matter in the practice of medicine: intelligence, fortitude, scientific acumen, compassion, dedication, leadership abilities, and communication skills. However, how do you put these all together into a cohesive and compelling narrative? How do you set yourself apart from the crowd without seeming like yet another cardboard applicant? Pay attention to the examples we include in this chapter of stellar candidates who built a fascinating story for themselves and followed their passion, rather than just checking boxes.

OK... so what are the qualities medical schools are looking for?

1. Intellectual ability

Medical school is sometimes characterized as "drinking from a fire hose." As a medical student, you are expected to learn a vast sum of information in an infinitesimal amount of time. This deluge of things to know will pile up relentlessly, like being forced to stand on the shore as tidal waves crash upon you without end. The information will often be difficult to conceptualize, memorize and integrate, and at some schools you will be graded and ranked against your (brilliant) classmates on a curve. As a physician, you will be expected to appraise a clinical situation quickly and with great comprehension, so you can apply your medical knowledge appropriately and effectively. This must be done despite being possibly fatigued and overworked to an extreme degree. A person may be compassionate, may be motivated, and may be tireless; all of those traits are important (and admirable), but if he or she is not particularly bright, they will struggle to be a successful physician.

One may argue whether classroom ability is an accurate reflection of one's intellectual prowess, but there's no way around it: your academic record during your undergraduate years in college does matter.

Your collegiate performance has two main dimensions: How challenging was your curriculum, and how well did you perform?

Box 2: What data do med schools think is most important when assessing an applicant?

An AAMC study of 142 admissions deans, committee members, and staff at 113 medical schools across the U.S. and Canada were asked to rank what they consider most important when choosing whom to invite to interview for a spot at their medical schools. Here are the averaged results in descending order of importance.[1]

Scale:
5: Extremely Important
4: Very Important
3: Important
2: Somewhat Important
1: Not important

Results:
Science GPA (sGPA): **3.7**
Cumulative GPA (cGPA): **3.6**
MCAT total score: **3.5**
Letters of recommendation: **3.4**
Clinical volunteering: **3.3**
Personal statements: **3.2**
Clinical work experience: **3.2**
Non-clinical volunteering: **3.1**
Leadership experience: **3.0**
Meeting pre-med requirements: **3.0**
Experience with the underserved: **2.7**

We consider both. For instance, we evaluate whether you chose an easier curriculum and excelled with little effort, or whether you pursued a challenging curriculum and performed well in spite of it. To that end, we look at many things, including your cumulative grade point average (GPA), your science GPA, your choice of major, the classes you took, the heft of your course load, and what college you attended. These considerations are not weighted equally and are holistically taken into consideration—in other words, we consider them all together to form a bigger picture.

1a. Your cumulative GPA

The most important measure of your academic performance is, ultimately, your cumulative GPA (cGPA). We value candidates' GPAs because they are a sustained and longitudinal record of an applicant's long-term motivation and academic ability. This is not only our opinion but also a prevailing one among other admissions officers throughout the country—and it shows: From 2017 to 2020, 65.5% of applicants with a 3.8-4.0 GPA were accepted to at least one allopathic (MD) medical school, while only 16.1% of those with a 3.0-3.19 GPA had the same outcome.[2] For medical school matriculants in 2018-2019, the average cGPA was a 3.72—or about an A- average.[3] The average GPA has been rising incrementally every year since 2001, when the same figure was a 3.60 GPA, according to the AAMC.[4] It is worth noting that these figures and probabilities vary with respect to the ethnicity of the applicant. For more on race and admissions, see Chapter 12.

1b. Your science GPA

We like to examine a candidate's science classes in particular. All of a candidate's biology, chemistry, physics, and mathematics (BCPM) course grades are computed to form the science GPA (sGPA).

Figure 1: Percentage accepted into a medical school by GPA, 2010-2012 (AAMC), N= 80,375

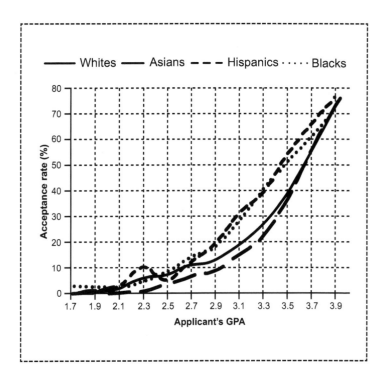

If an applicant has a poor sGPA, this may alert us that the candidate may not be very good at the sort of abilities that are necessary to excel in a science course—like mathematical and analytical reasoning. These are the same skills necessary in medicine, because so much of medicine is applied science. As such, a candidate with a good cGPA may be undermined by a poor sGPA. The same 2018-2019 med school matriculants had an average sGPA of 3.65.[5]

1c. Your course load

Most admissions officers want to get an idea of how rigorous and difficult an applicant's classes have been throughout college. That may include examining the course titles and whether they are upper (graduate) vs. lower level classes, as well as looking at the number of units taken per semester as a function of course load.

That being said, a transcript may be misleading, or not tell the whole story. The transcript lists the title of the class and the department to which the class belongs, but often not a whole lot more than that. As an example, let's say Physics 101 and 105 are both introductory classes, but 105, in reality, is much more difficult because it is calculus-based while 101 is not. An admissions officer may or may not have a way of telling the two apart unless she happens to be quite knowledgeable about the university that offers those courses. Thus, she may very well view both equally, even though an "A" grade in 105 may be much harder to earn than in 101. As a result, applicants who opt to take Physics 101 may end up with a higher GPA and have more time to pursue valuable extracurriculars, leading to a more impressive application than those who take 105.

So what matters more: a higher GPA with a somewhat lighter course load and easier classes, or a slightly lower GPA that resulted from more rigorous coursework? This is not an easy or straightforward question to answer. From the example above, you may think it's possible to 'game' the system in your favor and get your 4.0 while not having to challenge yourself unnecessarily...but be warned, you proceed along this path at your own peril. First of all, if you take this "softer" approach during your undergraduate studies, will you be as well-conditioned to handle the ramp-up of rigorous coursework if you do make it into medical school one day? And secondly: you never know whether someone sitting on the admissions committee just may be an alumnus of your school, and calls out your application (and, by association, you) for taking the easier path to a higher GPA. We've seen that precise situation occur—and it severely damaged that candidate's chances. On the other hand, we've also seen students take on a heavy course load, possibly even double major, only to end up with a mediocre cGPA, possibly with a few C's, and not get into medical school because their cGPA was too low for even consideration.

Our general advice is to take a more rigorous course load only if you can maintain a cGPA of 3.72 and sGPA of 3.65. As noted above, these are the averages for medical school matriculants in 2018-2019.

1d. Your GPA trajectory

We all cheer on the underdog who struggles at the beginning only to rally to victory at the end. Admissions officers are spectators to the performance of undergraduates in the same manner. We like to see students who recover from a poor early undergraduate performance and manage to finish the second half of their college career on a high note. A poor freshman year can be redeemed by a strong performance in later years, especially if the curriculum is difficult. Of course, it is better to have a consistently strong record all four years than it is to only have a strong record in the final one or two. Conversely, a downward trajectory is worrisome and may demonstrate a lack of motivation or stamina. Such a performance is a red flag and will require an explanation, like extenuating circumstances such as a sustained illness or serious financial problems. Any grades of C, D or—heaven forbid—F will give pause to admissions committee members. If you have any of these on your transcript—or an incomplete grade (I) or a withdrawal (W)—be prepared to explain why. On a similar note, it is fine to take an occasional course without a letter grade (a pass/fail grading system), but a widespread pattern of pass/fail classes will raise eyebrows. Note that all pre-requisite medical school courses must be taken for a letter grade.

1e. Your choice of major

Related to course load is your choice of major. In general, some majors are more challenging than others by reputation, with the average GPA being historically lower for those majors. A 3.8 GPA in mechanical engineering, for example, will likely be viewed more favorably than a 4.0 GPA in a traditionally easier major, like communications or psychology (not to disparage those majors). That being said, we encourage you to pursue a major you find most interesting. College is an unparalleled opportunity to learn about a wide range of topics from the best minds in the world, and we believe you should seize the opportunity to learn the subjects that intrigue you most. You can be accepted into medical school with any major, science or non-science. We find that when people study what they love, they are more motivated and perform better. Only pursue a double major if you are genuinely passionate about both fields of interest, not because you are trying to impress.

As mentioned, it is better to have a 3.8 GPA with a single major than struggling to maintain a 3.3 with a double major.

Figure 2: Entering 2019 Class Profile by Undergraduate Major- University of Michigan School of Medicine, N= 7, 896

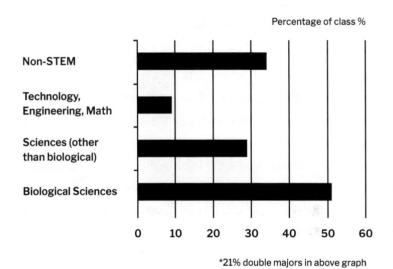

*21% double majors in above graph

1f. Your undergraduate institution

One of the cold realities of life is that the thin veneer of beauty and prestige is often taken more seriously than the content and character that lies beneath. Just as a Gucci and Prada purse will always don a higher price tag than a lesser-brand purse of equal fabric and quality, so too will an elite school be more highly valued over a 2nd tier university, no matter its quality of instruction. While we find great applicants from so-called lesser schools, the truth is that name brand and recognition do carry some clout, and so candidates from Ivy League and comparable institutions may have some (arguably unfair) advantages.

Added to this fact is that top-ranked medical schools will recruit heavily, and look more favorably, upon candidates from their own undergraduate institutions. At elite medical schools, it is not uncommon for over three-quarters of the interviewees at interview day to be from a top-20 undergraduate institution.

If you're on the outside looking in, don't despair, but at the same time be realistic. Applicants from more modest schools who do get in to a highly ranked medical school tend to have an ace in their sleeve, like being a university medalist (i.e., "valedictorian"), a high-score superstar (MCAT>524), or having a hobby, interest, or background that sets them apart (e.g., a combat medic veteran, a concert musician, or a varsity athlete). If you have none of these but are still an excellent applicant, it may be worth it to take a shot at few "dream" schools. After all, who knows how your application may somehow uniquely appeal to someone on that school's admissions committee? But reserve some energy and efforts on lower- to medium-tiered institutions and remember that in the end, you'll still come out with that M.D. degree.

1g. Summary

- A strong GPA is absolutely essential; make sure this remains a high (if not *the* highest) priority for you as an undergraduate student.

- A poor science GPA can undermine an overall strong GPA.

- A rigorous course load, jobs, a challenging major, a reputable school, and extensive extracurricular involvement can make a strong GPA even more attractive or can *slightly* compensate for a modest GPA.

- A poor GPA can benefit from an upward trend, just as a good GPA can be tarnished by a downward one.

- Even a student from a lower-ranked undergraduate school can become a strong medical school applicant—but may have to prove their academic prowess and exceptional abilities more than others

2. Passion for helping others

Every year there are amazing applicants who don't get in. One common reason is that—while they may have off-the-chart GPAs, MCAT scores, and stellar research experience—they provide insufficient evidence that they genuinely want to serve other people.

Doctors are, first and foremost, healers who are tasked

with the tremendous responsibility of maintaining and saving the most precious things of all: people's health, and often life itself. While the human body may be a machine of sorts, the physician who services the body is much more than a mere mechanic. Doctors who understand that their life's work is *people* and not *bodies* will find their jobs significantly more rewarding, and, by respecting their patients, will go the extra mile to care for them. When a patient is excellently cared for, his or her health outcomes are much more likely to be better. As admissions committee members, we want candidates who appreciate the joy that comes from serving others, who demonstrate a real passion for helping others, and who possess evidence of empathy and compassion.

Box 3: Volunteering and work examples for pre-med students

Volunteering (more altruistic)

• Sports for the physically and mentally handicapped
• Geriatric and dementia day care centers and clinics
• Mentoring programs and summer camps for disabled or under-served youths
• Teaching your skills (music, computers, drawing, etc.) to a dis-advantaged population for free
• Free community health clinics
• Hospice care centers
• Shelters for the homeless or victims of domestic violence
• Prisoner rehabilitation programs
• Hospital volunteering (try out more than one department, and choose clinical over nonclinical positions)
• Working for local charity groups, humanitarian organizations, and non-governmental organizations (NGOs)
• Multi-year service organizations, like Peace Corps and Teach for America—see chapter 4, "Gap Years"

Work (earns money)

• Phlebotomist (collection of blood samples)
• Basic emergency medical technician (EMT), ~3-5 month com-mitment to certify
• Certified nursing assistant (CNA)
• Hospital patient transporter
• Emergency department (ED) scribe: A physician's personal as-sistant and documentarian
• Electrocardiogram (ECG) technician
• Research assistant and tutoring (can be unpaid volunteering, too)

There are many ways to demonstrate these qualities, both within medicine and outside of it. The most com-petitive applicants tend to pursue sustained, long-term volunteering experiences in both clinical and non-clin-ical environments, as we will discuss in the following examples. While it may seem natural to pursue activi-ties within a clinical setting to gain valuable experience interacting directly with patients, don't assume this is the end-all/be-all. In fact, if you find yourself with the opportunity and drive to serve others in some other context that is not directly medical related, whether local or global, then we encourage you to go for it; such experiences may serve you just as well in your future career as a physician.

Just as a warning: during the application and interview phase, don't overplay your accomplishments or seem fake or uninspired in your desire to help others. There is nothing more appalling (and ironic) than exaggerating your accounts of altruism in an attempt to edge out your competitors.

2a. Clinical volunteering

Clinical volunteering is great in that it not only allows you to serve others, but it also allows you to do so while exposing you to what medicine is really all about, and a chance to decide if medicine is a good fit for you.

Medicine is a diverse field of practice, taking on many forms, and, as a result, so too is clinical volunteering. This kind of volunteerism can be quite traditional, like participating at a hospital, a private practice, or a neighborhood clinic. It can also be surprisingly unusual, like volunteering at sporting and musical events to assist attendees and performers who get hurt. The common thread in any kind of clinical volunteering is close, *personal interaction with patients*. Find out what you are passionate about, and volunteer in an interest related to that passion. For instance, if you enjoy the company of the elderly or have had loved ones with dementia, you may find it rewarding to volunteer at an Alzheimer's clinic. If you enjoy spending time with children, consider volunteering at a pediatric clinic or a summer camp for disabled youths.

A common pitfall among pre-meds is to pursue unfulfilling volunteer experiences at local hospitals. Many of these hospitals are in college towns, and, as a result, have volunteer programs that are saturated with premeds like you. These programs tend to suffer a high turnover rate, as students feel they are placed into volunteer positions that are not clinical or are unfulfilling and trivial (i.e., delivering X-rays, cleaning rooms, or manning the gift shop). If you are in this situation, get out! Find other experiences that give you more autonomy and meaningful patient interaction. Local free clinics and hospice care centers often give volunteers more responsibilities and opportunities for patient interaction.

Of special note, recognize that some forms of clinical volunteering may require special training and certification, such as first aid/basic life support or emergency medical technician (EMT) certification. Due to this extra training, these positions may give a volunteer much more responsibility and a direct hands-on role in providing medical treatment. These certifications can also be used to get a paid job in an entry-level medical field. Be warned, however, that these certifications may also require a considerable amount of time and often a hefty sum of money—and this may not be a worthwhile price compared to the importance of spending time studying to maintain the all-important GPA.

Whatever you choose, focus your volunteering efforts on activities that help others in a productive and meaningful way. Explore your community, network with peers and locals, and discover overlooked volunteering opportunities that exist around your community. Choose a position tailored to your interests where you will be useful. If you are not growing, learning, and having fun when you are volunteering, then you're probably doing it wrong!

2b. Non-clinical volunteering

While non-clinical volunteering may not give you exposure to the field of medicine, it demonstrates a commitment to others and, potentially, your local community. A useful aspect of non-clinical volunteering is that it is a broader field than clinical volunteering, with more opportunities and greater freedom to choose activities that match your particular interests. In the process, it may help set you apart in some unique fashion or shape your application in a positive way.

As such, non-clinical volunteering represents an opportunity to be creative and have fun. Do you enjoy playing music? Then volunteer your time playing for the elderly or the sick, or teach underprivileged children how to play your instrument of choice. Do you enjoy sports and games? Take some time to mentor a child through programs such as the Boys and Girls Club. Do you enjoy writing? Then volunteer to write for a publication that advocates for causes you support.

There are some activities that are considered top-tier by admissions officers that can significantly boost the strength of a candidate's application. These activities are usually quite long-term and demonstrate serious humanitarianism. Examples include the Peace Corps, Teach for America, or fieldwork with international NGOs (non-governmental organizations). These activities are typically pursued *after* undergraduate instruction, so we'll discuss them in Chapter 4 which covers "gap years"—a period of time some applicants take between their undergraduate and medical school years.

2c. Global volunteering

A common myth is that a top candidate must have volunteer experience overseas, usually in a "third-world" or developing nation. This is certainly not a requirement, though it can be a plus—or, believe it or not, potentially even a minus!

Students who pursue such activities often do so as part of a humanitarian relief group, their church, or some other organization, and they provide on-the-ground assistance in distributing supplies, performing administrative and clerical work, and unskilled manual aid. They often travel with other medical professionals who volunteer alongside them. The volunteers typically shadow and assist these professionals to a limited extent. We admire students who give up their money and comforts to help those in extreme poverty overseas, and we find these applicants often have unusual, eye-opening, and character-building experiences that they recount during interviews and in essays.

Be aware: there is a small but vocal minority of admissions officers who have issues with overseas volunteering.

They allege that such efforts can be exploitative, dangerous to patients, and are a privilege exclusive to wealthy pre-med students who can afford the expense of a transcontinental excursion.

In no way should you discuss your experiences with an air of condescension toward others ("oh, those poor, Dark Age tribal villagers…") or with an implied sense of disgust ("I couldn't believe we had to use squat toilets!").

Keep in mind that students who do not volunteer globally still have a myriad of opportunities to do meaningful, impactful volunteer work right at home. We appreciate candidates who serve the poor and underserved people who live right here in our local communities.

This is why global volunteering is in no way expected or required.

Box 4: How to find doctors to shadow

It's often daunting for pre-medical students to find a physician to shadow, especially if they have no family connections. A good first step is to utilize your family connections (if any), and ask your family doctor, especially if you have a long-standing relationship with him or her.

Another good way to find physicians is through a local major hospital, especially if it's a teaching hospital affiliated with a medical school. Academic physicians tend to be much more receptive to shadowing, and major hospitals have another key resource: an online faculty directory and a list of physicians on their hospital web site. We recommend compiling a list of physician names from the hospital web site, searching those names in the staff directory, and assembling a list of physician emails from the directory results. Then, send a concise and succinct e-mail to each physician in which you state your name, your school, your progress in school, and that you are interested in their field of practice and would like the shadowing.

In general, the vast majority of physicians are simply too busy to let a stranger shadow them. But if you email enough physicians, you are likely to find a handful willing to let you shadow them. Always be courteous and professional—remember, they are doing you a great favor. If a physician denies you, ask if they know any colleagues who will let you shadow. This extra question will increase your success rate dramatically.

It is best to email the physician directly, because calling can be too invasive, and phoning the office may lead you to a receptionist who may be unwilling to help you. Don't be afraid to be bold (but polite) when finding a physician to shadow. The rewards can be great when you succeed.

2d. Summary

- Clinical volunteering is a two-fold process of serving others while gaining valuable clinical exposure and insight.

- Volunteer work that requires some form of intensive training or medical certification can be incredibly valuable and lead to great clinical experiences. But be careful that they don't become too time-consuming and grade-destroying that they end up being counter-productive.

- Pursue volunteering that is unique, fun, meaning-ful, and relevant to your interests, whether clinical-ly-related or not. Network to find out interesting opportunities that are off the beaten path.

- Overseas volunteering is often impressive but by no means necessary. If you do it, don't do anything unethical.

---

3. Growth, commitment, and leadership

Your application is more than a laundry list of activi-ties. You are not trophy hunting. Your activities are a re-flection of what you've done, who you are, and what you value. Ideally, the activities you pursue in college reflect your growth as a person, exploration of the things that interest you, commitment to the organizations and ac-tivities you've enjoyed the most, and, eventually, lead-ership within those groups after long-standing partic-ipation. To emphasize, we like to see participants who have a clearly defined passion (or set of passions), a devel-opment of those interests through a logical set of activities, and growth and leadership within those activities.

These interests and activities, if coherent and *sustained*, form a thematic narrative that can be quite compelling. This narrative allows a candidate to stand out from other applicants who are often "cookie-cutter" and have an unoriginal, vague, incoherent, or underdeveloped set of interests and activities.

Try your best to understand what you are passionate about. If you aren't sure, go exploring and pursue a diverse set of interests to find out just what it is you like. Once you know, then be bold, creative, and original when it comes to fashioning your own set of extracurricular activities that reflect and complement what you like. After you do that, be sure to stick with those activities, develop them further, and take a creative, leading role within those activities. Rather than juggle a hundred disparate commitments at once, focus on a few that are important to you and stick with them. In these cases, quality is far better than quantity. Students who take on too many projects often find themselves spread too thinly and ruin their grades—which are just as important as volunteering, if not more.

Applicants who have faced personal challenges (e.g., a serious disability, financial ruin, the death of a parent) may be able to frame these events as opportunities for growth. For example, a candidate who loses a limb might become an organizational leader for others with similar disabilities. A candidate whose family hit financial rock-bottom may later spearhead a scholarship organization for poor and disadvantaged youths.

Athletes—especially varsity athletes—enjoy a particular

advantage in the admissions process. We are impressed by athletes who maintain good grades and get good MCAT scores while juggling the time-consuming demands of their sport. Competitive athletics also has inherent opportunities for growth, challenge, and leadership, all of which we admire.

Nontraditional applicants—such as athletes, the physically challenged, the economically or socially disadvantaged, military, and older candidates—often have unique characteristics, experiences, and opportunities for growth, which we will discuss further in Chapter 12.

Box 5: What separates a good extracurricular activity from a great one? An example of growth, commitment, and leadership.

Average: Volunteered once for 1 week as a counselor at a summer camp for disabled pre-teens.

Good: Did what was average, but also returned the next year and the year after that in the same capacity.

Great: Did what was good, and also organized a school-wide fundraiser to expand the quality and size of the summer camp program.

Outstanding: Did what was great, and also improved the activities at the camp, trained new counselors, and worked to create a new summer camp program for underserved children.

---

4. Exposure to medicine

If you're going to buy a $200 pair of shoes you intend on wearing for several years, then it's obvious you should try them on first to make sure they fit comfortably.

To become a doctor is like buying a If you're going to buy a $200 pair of shoes you intend on wearing for several years, then it's obvious you should try them on first to make sure they fit comfortably. To become a doctor is like buying a pair of shoes that cost $200,000+ that you'll wear for the rest of your working life. So, doesn't it make sense to "try it on" first? We like candidates who have ample exposure to the medical field and the life of a physician because it shows that they have tried it on, to an extent.

The best way to gain exposure to medicine is through clinical volunteering, as discussed above, and physician shadowing. We're not only looking for candidates who demonstrate altruism, we're also looking for applicants who have taken some time to see what it is like to be not only a health professional, but, more particularly, *a physician*. We recommend you pursue clinical activities that allow you to see directly what a doctor's day-to-day life is like. Shadowing is an effective way to achieve that end, because you get to follow a doctor while he practices medicine. Hospital volunteers often have this opportunity, if they are in the right position, like in the emergency room rather than the front desk of the hospital lobby.

We recommend you gain exposure to physicians of all kinds of practice. You'll find the day-to-day responsibilities of, say, an academic pathologist at a research-heavy urban medical school is far different than a rural family doctor at a private practice in an underserved community.

If you have a particular specialty, patient population, or lifestyle in mind, we recommend you follow a physician that matches what you envision for yourself as a doctor.

Another excellent way to "shadow" is to actually get paid to shadow—also known as scribing. Scribes follow emergency room doctors and act as their personal assistants. They may record the history of a patient's illness, document the physical examination, enter vital signs, look up medical records, keep track of imagining studies, type progress notes, and enter the patient's discharge plan. Call your local hospitals and ask if they have a scribe program. Many hospitals have contracts with private agencies that train and manage scribes.

---

5. Competence in the scientific method

Medicine is, at least partly, an applied science of biology, chemistry, and physics, and medical treatments are developed and refined by basic, clinical, translational, and epidemiological research. A good physician not only has a strong grasp of scientific concepts, but is also able to quickly understand and synthesize new scientific literature and apply it to improve how they practice medicine. Many physicians contribute to the field of medicine by producing their own research. We like to see candidates who possess not only an ability to understand science but also an appreciation and aptitude for the research that adds to our understanding of medicine.

Elite medical schools are home to billions of dollars of medical research. They aim to educate future physicians who will not only provide excellent patient care but also may contribute to advancing the field of medicine through original discovery. If you are at all interested in research or joining a top medical school, acquiring research experience in your undergraduate years is *virtually required.* Even if you do not attend a top school, most medical schools appreciate research experience. According to the AAMC, 92% of accepted applicants to Harvard Medical School had research experience. At the Creighton University School of Medicine—a less selective, Jesuit, patient-care centered school in Nebraska—83% of accepted students had research experience. Research is the norm, not the exception, regardless of the school to which you apply.

Like volunteering, we encourage you to choose a field of research that matches your interests and passions. While it probably makes the most sense to pursue research in a medically-related field, other avenues of research—whether it be applied physics, social psychology, or evolutionary biology—are also valuable and can be a tremendous boost to the quality of your application. We want to see that your research is sustained, in-depth and productive, no matter the subject.

When it comes to evaluating the quality of your research involvement, we look for signs that you had to use and hone the skills associated with scientific research: inquisitiveness, critical thinking, creativity, and persistence. The best candidates do much more than mindless manual labor for their principal investigator. They develop their own research projects, learn to work independently, and contribute to the intellectual work of their lab mates, whether through partnerships or feedback at lab meetings. A big plus is candidates who publish their research in scientific journals or present their findings on posters at research conferences, because it shows they have the skills necessary to produce a piece of work worthy of consideration by the scientific community, and that their lab finds their work worthy of endorsement. We also look at the position of your name in the list of authors of a poster or publication, because being closer to the front of the list implies you had greater role in the more intellectual aspects of research production, including experimental design, methods, data analysis, or writing the published work.

Box 6: How to find a good research position

It can be quite a task to find a laboratory willing to take you on as an undergraduate research assistant, even if the position is unpaid. You must be both persistent and bold when finding a good lab to join.

First, do your homework. Many universities have an undergraduate research apprenticeship program that acts as a matchmaker program for undergraduate students who are interested in getting their feet wet in research. These programs can be invaluable resources that do all the networking for you. The downside is that these programs tend to have more applicants than spaces, and only students with the best grades and credentials will likely get the coveted research positions.

Another option is to carve your own route. Use your college's website to find links to labs on campus, and use the faculty directory to get email addresses for the principal investigator (P.I., also known as the professor in charge of the lab), post-doctoral fellows (lab members with doctoral degrees), and graduate students (PhD and MA candidates). Find out the specific research they are currently working on. This is best done by reading their most recently published research papers. Note what you find interesting about their current research, then email whoever is working on that research. Tell them you are interested in meeting to discuss questions you had on their research, and how you would like to help them with it. If you can communicate your interest and how you can help them (and not how they can help you!), they will likely accept you into their lab with an entry-level position.

If this doesn't work, try and try again! Most colleges have countless labs, especially if you open yourself up to other subjects and disciplines. You can also find labs at nearby colleges, medical schools, and private research institutions (e.g., pharmaceutical and biotechnology companies) that may be receptive to help. If you know or are shadowing academic physicians, they may know a good clinical research opportunity for you. With hard work, passion and creativity, you can work your way up from mindless manual labor to doing intellectual, creative work of your own in a lab. And if you cannot progress, then, well, find a new lab!

The quality, prestige, and viewership of the journal in which you are published are sometimes considered, especially if the journal is particularly reputable (high impact score) and widely circulated.

Candidates who have a particular clinical interest often

pursue research and volunteering within that field. We like these applicants because they demonstrate a multifaceted commitment to one particular arena, which adds to their thematic narrative (see #3: "Growth, commitment, and leadership" in this chapter to revisit this concept).

Box 7: Do med schools care about your pre-college activities?

For many students, applying to medical school may seem like déjà vu. In many respects it is a familiar retread of applying to college while in high school. Like applying to med school, undergrad admissions requires a standardized national entrance exam, GPA, and extracurricular activities. So, it may seem to make some sense that the extracurricular activities that wooed your undergraduate admissions committee will do the same for the medical school committee.

In reality, most med school admissions faculty don't really care about what you did while you attended high school or middle school. Achievements or activities from high school are routinely glossed over by medical school admissions committees.

However, there are some exceptions. Clinical experiences, such as volunteering or shadowing, can be referenced in interviews and essays as part of your motivation for pursuing a career as a physician. Moreover, some admissions officers like seeing activities that demonstrate extraordinary achievement and multi-year dedication, like becoming an eagle scout or earning a black belt in a martial art at a young age. In other words, don't write down that you did karate in high school—unless you earned a black belt and won some superlative competitive award. Focus on college and post-college achievements.

For example, a pre-med student interested in health outcomes in developing nations may do epidemiological research on flu prevention among infants in the Haitian immigrant community in their hometown while volunteering at a local clinic that serves the same population.

Perhaps the student became interested in the research

after observing in the clinic that babies from first-generation immigrant homes were more likely to get the flu than those with second-generation parents. Intrigued by this higher incidence, the pre-med student is now interested in going to Haiti while in medical school to do research on whether these differential outcomes truly exist.

---

6. Integrity and professionalism

Doctors generally command a good deal of respect from the public partly because they are viewed as examples of virtue, trust, and expertise. A physician has tremendous responsibilities, and, as such, they should possess a great deal of integrity and professionalism. Poor judgment, aggressiveness, impulsiveness, arrogance, and a lack of genuineness are all bright red flags, and your record should never show any indication of these negative qualities.

Every year, we encounter students who show some sign of these unfortunate traits. Undergraduate college reports will list any misdeeds that an applicant may have committed. Some are excusable; others require a detailed explanation, while a few are virtually impossible to forgive. Felonies, repeated instances of cheating, and serious fabrications on applications will guarantee a zero chance of admission into medical school. Possession of alcohol in the dorms, an instance of plagiarism, or a misdemeanor are evaluated on a case-by-case basis, and your explanation of the circumstances can be key in our evaluation. Be contrite, demonstrate how you have learned from your mistakes, and explain how these actions are not indicative of a larger problem. If we discover you have withheld or suppressed evidence of an infraction of any kind—big or small—your application will be in serious jeopardy.

How much of all of this do I need to do?

In general, a strong applicant demonstrates every quality we have listed. Keep in mind that volunteering and research, while essential, should be limited to only as much as you can manage while still maintaining a strong GPA. Extracurricular activities can be more flexibly rescheduled, if necessary, to fit into your vacations, weekends, and after-hours, while it is much harder to re-take a class or compensate for a bad grade (i.e., a permanent, irrevocable blemish on your college transcript).

A common pre-med question is "how many hours do I need?" for research or volunteering. The answer is: it depends on how much time you need in order to be productive. We look more at results, achievements, and how long-term your involvement was, with an emphasis on the quality rather than the quantity of hours you spent. 200 hours pipetting into tubes without any creative work is less valuable than 50 hours designing your own experiment and getting published. Applicants to medical school typically have over 100 hours of clinical volunteering, research, and shadowing, with many candidates having significantly more than that. Many of these numbers do have diminishing returns. For example, while we like to see applicants who have shadowed for more than a few hours, we do not find it much more impressive to commit 100 hours to shadowing versus 300—both figures seem like more than enough to demonstrate that you have shadowed sufficiently.

Summary

Because so many people apply to medical school, not everyone can be accepted. Medical schools are quite selective because they can afford to be. To set yourself apart, your GPA, MCAT score, and extracurriculars must be excellent. Lacking in any of these may hamstring your chances of acceptance.

While all are important, some factors are more important than others for being admitted to medical school. In descending order of importance: GPA, MCAT score, clinical volunteering or work, non-clinical volunteering or work, and leadership experiences are considered. Make sure you keep your GPA and MCAT strong, more than anything.

> Research experience is especially important—and virtually required—if you intend on applying to a top-tier medical school. Find a research field you genuinely enjoy, as most fields of research will be valued by admissions committees.

---

[1] https://www.aamc.org/download/261106/data/aibvol11_no6.pdf

[2] https://www.aamc.org/system/files/2020-04/2019_FACTS_Table_A-23_0.pdf

[3] https://www.kaptest.com/study/mcat/whats-the-aveage-gpa-for-medical-school-matriculants/

[4] https://www.aamc.org/download/321494/data/2013factstable17.pdf

[5] https://www.kaptest.com/study/mcat/whats-the-aveage-gpa-for-medical-school-matriculants/

Figure 1:
https://www.aamc.org/data/facts/applicantmatriculant/157998/mcat-gpa-grid-by-selected-race-ethnicity.html

Figure 2:
https://medicine.umich.edu/medschool/sites/medicine.umich.edu.medschool/files/assets/Incoming%20Class%20of%202019.pdf

Chapter III

The Medical College Admission Test (MCAT)

For many aspiring medical students, especially those who are not fans of test-taking (and really, who is?), there is no larger impediment to entering medical school than the MCAT. While you may be familiar with another standardized test—the SAT—the MCAT is a longer and more arduous entrance exam. With fierce competition to enter medical school, the MCAT often serves as a "first cut" at many institutions to weed out students who are less likely to be successful at handling the academic rigors of medical school. Even at one of the least selective medical schools in the nation, the class of 2023 had an average MCAT score of 509—a performance better than 79 percent of all test-takers.[1]

A low score often (but not always) can sink an applicant's chances, as some admissions officers consider

MCAT scores to be about as paramount as GPA when deciding whom to invite to interview. For some pre-med students, precious time, mental energy, and money is spent taking and retaking the exam in an attempt to achieve a score that will make them competitive for medical school admission.

That being said, there is a ray of light among the clouds. The good news is, with *lots of well-planned* studying, most applicants can earn a competitive MCAT score, while other graduate school exams are resistant to improvement despite intensive study. In this chapter, we will discuss the strategies that are most conducive toward success on the MCAT.

1. What is the MCAT, exactly?

As described in the *Flexner Report*, American medical schools were once far less selective and had no entrance examinations. At the dawn of the 20th century, many wishing to become a doctor could "walk into a medical school from the street" and some "could barely read and write." By the 1920s, dropout rates from American medical colleges reached 50 percent.[2] A prototype of the MCAT—the Scholastic Aptitude Test for Medical Students—was devised to ensure medical schools only admitted students who had the academic capacity to survive the intense intellectual rigor of medical school.

By 1948, the test was renamed "MCAT" and became multiple choice. By 1992, the MCAT resembled the test that we had up until 2015[3] In 2015, the AAMC unveiled a new MCAT, which it optimistically titles "MCAT2015: A Better Test for Tomorrow's Doctors" (yes, that is a superscript). Unlike the earlier versions of the test, the current exam gauges more than factual knowledge; it also assesses conceptual understanding and critical thinking. It tests college-level, introductory-level concepts in general chemistry, physics, biology, organic chemistry, and verbal reasoning in a timed, computerized format. Think of AP Physics, AP Chemistry, AP Biology, and AP English tests amalgamated into one super-exam.

MCAT subjects are grouped into four sections as described below:

Table 1: 2015-Present MCAT Format:

Section	Score range	#Questions	Minutes
Biological and Biochemical Foundations of Living Systems:	118 to 132	59	95
Chemical and Physical Foundations of Biological Systems:	118 to 132	59	95
Psychological, Social, and Biological Foundations of Behavior:	118 to 132	59	95
Critical Analysis and Reasoning Skills:	118 to 132	53	90

The MCAT's sections are a tossed salad of multiple subjects, with significant subject overlap between sections, recognizing that much of the practice and learning of medicine cannot be neatly compartmentalized. For instance, general biology, biochemistry, general chemistry, and organic chemistry now appear in two separate sections instead of just one self-contained section.[4] For a list of topics covered in each subject on the MCAT, visit the AAMC website.

Figure 1: Composition of each section by subject, MCAT

Biological and Biochemical Foundations of Living Systems	Chemical and Physical Foundations of Biological Systems	Psychological, Social, and Biological Foundations of Behavior

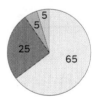 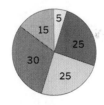 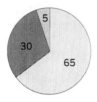

Biology: 65%
Biochemistry: 25%
General chemistry: 5%
Organic chemistry: 5%

General chemistry: 30%
Biochemistry: 25%
Physics: 25%
Organic chemistry: 15%
Biology: 5%

Psychology: 65%
Sociology: 30%
Biology: 5%

_____

1a. Scoring

The MCAT score range is 472 to 528 and is based on a curve. In other words, a test taker's score does not depend on how many questions he or she missed. Rather, it is based on how well they performed on the questions relative to how others did on the same questions. The AAMC constantly creates new sets of questions for the MCAT, so no one MCAT exam is the same as another. As a result, some exams end up more difficult than others. To ensure fairness among test takers, the AAMC calculates the difficulty of an exam based on performance among test takers, and it will then boost—or lower—test takers' scores based on how difficult the questions were. This ensures that any given score reflects a student's ability relative to his or her peers, rather than how easy that particular test happened to be.

_____

1b. What is a "good score?"

There are a couple of ways to look at this. Each MCAT score tracks to an approximate percentile rank, which is a measure of how many test takers achieve a higher score than you did. A percentile rank score of 99.0 means you have scored higher than 99% of the other test takers (that would be considered pretty good, in case you are wondering).

A good score is, moreover, one that is historically competitive for the school you desire to enter. By looking at the average MCAT scores of students previously accepted to that school, you can ascertain the score you need to be at least competitive for admission. In Table 2, we've listed median MCAT scores for accepted applicants to medical schools in 2019. Achieving a similar (or higher) MCAT score as a given medical school's average is ideal to be competitive for entry into that school. Keep in mind, GPA, interviews, extracurricular activities, letters of recommendation, and life circumstances and hardships will also be considered. In Figure 2, we show the percentage of applicants accepted to at least one medical school for each major ethnicity of applicants. As you can see, race can be a significant factor that affects your chances of getting into medical school (See Chapter XII). In Figure 3, we show the percentage of applicants who were accepted to at least one medical school by MCAT score and GPA.

Table 2: Estimated MCAT Percentile Rank Scores with School Averages

MCAT score	Percentile rank	Approximate accepted applicant average score (2019)
528	100	The University of Impossibly High Standards
522	99	NYU, Johns Hopkins
521	98	UPenn, Columbia, Wash U in St. Louis
519	97	Duke, Harvard, Stanford...
517	94	Boston U, UCLA, USC...
514	89	Dartmouth, Emory, Tufts, SUNY...
508	74	Texas Tech, East Carolina, Michigan State...
504	60	D.O. schools (Doctor of Osteopathy)
500	46	Lower-tier D.O. schools
496	33	Podiatry schools ("foot doctors")
491	20	None applicable.
486	10	None applicable.
477	1	None applicable.
475	<1	None applicable.
472	<1	None applicable.

Figure 2: Percentage accepted into a medical school by MCAT, 2010-2012 (AAMC), N=80,375

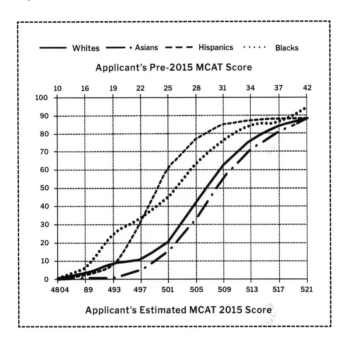

Encouragingly, although an excellent score is usually required to enter an MD school, one can still become a practicing physician with a below-average MCAT score. If you look at the graph, a small proportion of applicants with MCAT scores in the mid- to upper-20s still get admitted somewhere. There are also alternative routes you could pursue: Doctor of Osteopathy (DO) schools tend to have somewhat lower standards for admission, while individuals with even lower MCAT scores may still be competitive for podiatry school.

Figure 3: Percentage & Number of Applicants Accepted to One or More Medical Schools (2017-2019)

dark shading = ≥ 75% acceptance rates, medium shading = 50-74% acceptance rates, light shading = 25-49% acceptance rates

—

dashes: cells with > 10 observations, blank: cells with 0 observation

MCAT / GPA	472-485	486-489	490-493	494-497	498-501	502-505	506-509	510-513	514-517	518-528	All
3.80-4.00	3% 4/159	3% 9/320	8% 58/726	19% 298/1,584	31% 1,007/3,272	49% 2,603/5,435	62% 4,945/7,957	75% 6,573/8,778	82% 6,312/7,711	88% 6,893/7,848	66% 28,702/43,790
3.60-3.79	1% 3/382	1% 8/613	4% 55/1,313	12% 300/2,492	24% 1,017/4,251	35% 2,181/6,291	50% 3,770/7,565	65% 4,670/7,228	74% 3,526/4,793	81% 2,364/2,924	47% 17,894/37,852
3.40-3.59	1% 5/570	1% 10/846	3% 53/1,593	10% 266/2,683	19% 748/4,023	26% 1,340/5,059	37% 2,034/5,472	51% 2,290/4,497	62% 1,552/2,494	70% 881/1,252	32% 9,179/28,489
3.20-3.39	<1% 1/705	1% 6/835	2% 35/1,474	7% 155/2,183	15% 424/2,821	22% 683/3,176	30% 865/2,921	40% 865/2,170	51% 571/1,123	57% 252/443	22% 3,857/17,851
3.00-3.19	<1% 3/777	1% 7/743	2% 17/1,030	7% 94/1,433	14% 226/1,596	21% 327/1,591	25% 359/1,411	34% 339/1,004	41% 168/408	50% 100/201	16% 1,640/10,194
2.80-2.99	1% 5/673	1% 3/549	2% 14/659	4% 30/700	9% 67/756	17% 126/737	23% 132/565	27% 86/324	28% 48/169	41% 24/58	10% 535/5,190
2.60-2.79	0% 0/468	1% 4/320	1% 2/396	3% 11/354	8% 34/401	16% 44/267	18% 33/186	19% 21/113	40% 23/57	33% 6/18	7% 178/2,580
2.40-2.59	0% 0/331	1% 1/176	2% 3/175	5% 8/170	4% 5/124	13% 12/93	25% 17/69	26% 12/46	25% 4/16	–	5% 64/1,206
2.20-2.39	0% 0/194	0% 0/96	0% 0/83	3% 2/61	11% 5/44	21% 8/39	16% 5/32	14% 3/21	–	–	5% 29/579
2.0-2.19	0% 0/107	0% 0/30	3% 1/29	0% 0/20	–	8% 1/13	–	–	–	–	1% 3/221
<2.00	0% 0/51	7% 1/14	7% 1/14	0% 0/10	–	–	–	–	–	–	2% 2/94
All	<1% 21/4,417	1% 49/4,542	3% 239/7,492	10% 1,164/11,690	20% 3,533/17,297	32% 7,325/22,703	46% 12,160/26,187	61% 14,859/24,186	73% 12,209/16,779	83% 10,524/12,753	42% 62,083/148,046

2. How to prepare for the MCAT

The MCAT is not an IQ test, nor is it purely a measure of your inherent cognitive skills. What separates successful test takers from failed ones is unlikely to just be differences in intellect; rather, it has much to do with differences in study strategy.

2a. Early preparation

For students still in college, there are two common times to prepare for the MCAT—the summer after sophomore year or the summer after junior year. This allows them to focus on the MCAT when classes are over. Taking the MCAT by the end of junior year allows applicants enough time to apply to medical school during their senior year and enter a few months after graduating college. What many students do not realize is that preparation really begins right when you commence taking your first pre-med class. The MCAT is a test of topics covered in introductory-level college courses in the natural sciences, so it is essential that you do well and learn in your entry-level science courses. These include introductory courses in general chemistry (2 semesters), organic chemistry (1-2 semesters), physics (2 semesters), and general biology

(2 semesters), as well as 1-semester courses in bio-chemistry, statistics, psychology, and sociology.

It is not enough to simply earn an "A" in these courses to pad your science GPA. To do well on the MCAT, you should strive to do more than memorize the material the night before the midterm and final exams only to regurgitate the material on test day and quickly forget it thereafter in a haze of post-exam partying. Nerdy as it may sound, try to gain a deep conceptual understanding of the subject while you learn it. Whenever possible, figure out how subjects interrelate rather than viewing them as independent of one another. Know the material well enough to explain it well to both your classmates and your parents.

We recommend keeping detailed notes on your text-book reading assignments and lectures; they will make good review material for the MCAT, and the act of writing will help solidify what you've learned. Many students find it helpful to do sample MCAT problems while they take a relevant class – for example, doing a few physics problems each week while taking an introductory physics class.

_____

2b. Planning D-Day

When to schedule the test can be quite important to your success, in terms of what time of day, where the test is taken, and what time of year. Choose a test time that matches with your circadian rhythms, when you tend to be the most alert and fresh. Choose a location that is familiar and close by. Unfortunately, test dates fill up fast, so you must reserve your space early in order to maximize your freedom of choice (usually at least 60 days before your desired date). Note that the test is not offered every month of the year and occurs most frequently in the summer months. It takes about 30 days to receive a score after finishing the exam, so definitely plan to take the exam at least one month before you intend on applying to medical school so your score is ready by the time you submit your application. If you plan to turn in your primary application on or near opening day (early June), which is an ideal time, you should schedule your exam no later than early May...assuming, of course, that you will be satisfied with your score and do not need to re-take the exam.

Most students aim to take the test in the summer, when they tend to have fewer or no classes. Because MCAT studying should be intensive, try to carve out some dedicated time when you are not taking classes (or do not have a heavy course load). If you have already graduated and are working full-time, it may not always be possible to take time off, but explaining your situation to your employer may give you more flexibility in your work hours for at least a period of time. For those of you who are able to limit outside obligations, and if logistically and financially possible, plan to study diligently for

2-3 consecutive months prior to taking the MCAT. For others who may be limited to studying on nights and weekends because of full-time work or other circumstances, that time frame may be twice as long.

2c. MCAT preparatory classes versus self-study

There are two main ways to prepare for the test: alone or in a classroom format. While either approach can achieve good results, the question is which is right for you. If you need the structure and motivation of studying with others, a classroom format may be the best. If you feel weighed down by others and want to customize how you learn, it may be wiser to study alone.

If you choose to take a class, there are many test preparation companies that specialize in the MCAT and offer classroom instruction packaged with homework and practice materials. These courses offer a strict schedule of assignments, lectures, and practice tests to methodically assess and build your skills. The most popular brands are Kaplan, The Princeton Review, Examkrackers, Blueprint, and The Berkeley Review. These classes typically cost two to three thousand dollars, last anywhere from 1-6 months, and usually meet several times a week (often at night) for a few hours per session. Many companies offer hybridized or exclusive Internet courses where instructors offer feedback through the web.

If you elect to work alone, the same companies offer self-study guides that include content review material, practice problems, and mock exams, although you do not have access to the same range and extent of materials as you would if you enrolled in their class. A full set of new books may range from $200 to $700. One advantage of self-study is that you can mix and match the brands of books, as some companies may be better at some subjects than others. You also have more flexibility in choosing when and what to study, compared to taking a strictly regimented class; although self-paced online courses are beginning to offer the same advantage as self-studying but with the added resources of an online infrastructure and a burgeoning electronic database of practice questions.

Typically, the Examkrackers brand tends to be the most topical and easiest of the review books. On the other end of the spectrum, the Berkeley Review books are considered by many to be the most in-depth and difficult.

No matter which method you elect to pursue, be sure to occasionally take practice tests throughout your study schedule, especially right before the date of your official exam. Use early practice tests to identify weak spots in your understanding, and use later practice exams to hone your time-management skills and predict your performance on the real MCAT. If, by the end of your preparation, you consistently score below your desired score on your practice exams, it may behoove you to postpone your MCAT test date.

Remember: you cannot erase a poor official MCAT score from your record, and most medical schools consider all of your MCAT scores—not just the highest or most recent. Like diamonds, your MCAT score is forever.

2d. Stress, nerves, and rash decisions

While the MCAT is an academic test that measures your scholastic performance, it is also an exam that tests your coping abilities. The reality is about 70% of test takers will earn a score that is below-average for applicants accepted to medical school, and that fact dictates how difficult and stressful it can be for many applicants to prepare for and take the MCAT. Because the MCAT requires such intensive and prolonged study, it rewards applicants who exhibit determination, discipline, and self-confidence—all valuable traits for those who eventually go on to practice medicine. Sadly, for some, the stress of the exam is simply too much, and they fall off their study regimen, get distracted, or panic during the exam. Too many aspiring medical students decide that the MCAT is an impassable roadblock, and prematurely give up their dreams of becoming a physician.

The best antidote to test anxiety is to go into the exam as well-prepared as you possibly can, practicing frequently under timed conditions so you know how to pace yourself during the test, and not psych yourself out with a gloom-and-doom mentality. If you have studied diligently beforehand, begin the test knowing you did everything you could to optimize your chances of success and let the chips fall where they may. And, of course, make sure to get a good night's sleep beforehand!

---

3. Voiding scores and retaking the exam

At the end of the MCAT exam, you have the option of canceling your test *before* it is submitted to be graded. If you choose to void your exam, you will not receive a score, nor will medical schools be made aware of your decision to cancel the exam. Voiding the exam should only be done if you are *certain* you performed poorly. Many applicants—especially those who tend to be cautious or anxious—often underestimate their performance and run the risk of canceling a good score.

If you've received a low score, you have the option of retaking the exam, which can be taken a maximum of three times per year. Medical schools tend to view an applicant's multiple MCAT scores in the following ways:

- All scores are considered and weighed the same, and attention is paid to upward or downward trends (*most common*).

- Only the most recent score is considered.

- Only the highest score is considered.

- The average of all the scores is considered.

- The highest individual section scores are combined and considered.

Because most schools either average all the scores or consider them all holistically, there are risks to re-taking the exam, especially if you score the same or lower the second time around. Even a modest improvement on the re-take may not be particularly impressive, because the boost may be interpreted simply as a reflection of your greater experience taking the exam rather than your aptitude.

On the other hand, if you do perform significantly better on a retake, that can strengthen your application greatly; perhaps the first time around, there were extenuating circumstances, you had a bad case of nerves...or you may simply not have prepared adequately. Moreover, a willingness to take the test a second time around—and all the stress and preparation that goes into it—is an indication that you have both perseverance and a desire to improve, rather than just being satisfied with a sub-par score.

Figure 4: Changes in MCAT score for same year retests (AAMC)

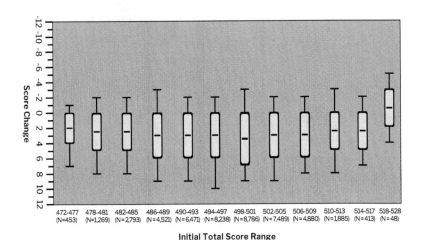

If you do decide to re-take the exam, identify what went wrong on the original attempt and only re-take the exam when you're confident it won't be repeated. Focus on the subsections you struggled with the most the first time around. As a general rule of thumb, if you've already scored well above 509 with your first attempt, there may not be tremendous value gained in retaking it just to add a few additional points to your score. One possible exception is if you score 125 or lower in any subsection, which some schools will view as an indictment of your verbal or scientific analytic skills.

The graph above from the AAMC displays how well test takers did on re-take exams from 2015-2017 based on their original score. Generally, the lower your original score, the more likely you are to gain a higher score on a re-take. The graph shows range, upper and lower quartiles, and the median for each MCAT score range.

Summary

- The MCAT is an entrance examination required for admittance to medical school, and it tests your knowledge of the pre-medical science courses you took in college, including general biology, chemistry, biochemistry, organic chemistry, physics, sociology, and psychology.

- Your performance on the MCAT can make or break your chances of getting into medical school. The median MCAT score of the least selective M.D. schools is in the 75th percentile—roughly speaking, their students tended to score better than about 75% of test-takers.

- The MCAT is perhaps the greatest barrier to entry to medical school, so it will require your determination, hard work, and careful planning. Preparing ahead, giving yourself ample study time, following a thoughtful study schedule, and using tutors or MCAT-prep services can greatly improve your score. While you study for the MCAT, get rid of distractions, and rely on friends and family to help support you through the challenges you may encounter during your preparation.

[1] https://medicine.hsc.wvu.edu/md-admissions/2023-class-profile/

[2] http://www.carnegiefoundation.org/sites/default/files/elibrary/Carn-egie_Flexner_Report.pdf, pg 22

[3] http://en.wikipedia.org/wiki/Medical_College_Admission_Test

[4] https://www.aamc.org/students/services/343550/mcat2015.html

Table 1:

https://www.aamc.org/students/applying/mcat/mcat2015/testsec-tions/

Figure 1:

https://students-residents.aamc.org/applying-medical-school/arti-cle/whats-mcat-exam/

Table 2:

https://aamc-orange.global.ssl.fastly.net/production/media/filer_public/d9/04/d904b7f4-c3d0-4469-aed1-e5afff500d05/mcat-to-tal_and_section_score_percentile_ranks_2020_for_web.pdf

https://www.usnews.com/education/best-graduate-schools

top-medical-schools/slideshows/10-med-schools-with-the-highest-mcat-scores?slide=24

Figure 2:

https://www.aamc.org/data/facts/applicantmatriculant/157998/mcat-gpa-grid-by-selected-race-ethnicity.html

Figure 3:

https://www.aamc.org/system/files/c/2/462316-mcatguide.pdf, Table 2

Figure 4:

https://www.aamc.org/system/files/c/2/462316-mcatguide.pdf, Fig 11

Chapter IV

Gap Years

W hat was traditional is now, increasingly, non-traditional. In the past, most students began medical school right after finishing their undergraduate education. But now, at some schools, a majority of students have taken at least one year off—and sometimes many more—before starting medical school. This time off between undergraduate and medical school is so common among applicants that it has its own name: the "gap years." These gap years can be a valuable asset to an applicant's chances of getting accepted to a medical school of their choice, depending on what they do during those years. Conversely, if that time is spent unproductively, it may raise a red flag and be a detriment to a candidate's application. In this chapter, we will discuss why applicants take gap years, what they do during these years, and how to make the most out of them.

Why students take gap years

Applicants come from all walks of life, and their reasons for taking gap years are equally as varied. Some students may be entirely ready and qualified to get into medical school right away, but wish to take time off to pursue some outside passion (which may be health-care-related or not), earn extra money to help with medical school tuition, or simply take a breather before diving into the rigors of medical training. For these applicants, a gap year or two may improve their already-competitive chances, sometimes to a significant degree if they are particularly productive during their time off, and we generally encourage this approach. Oftentimes, additional life experience makes for a more interesting, mature, and well-rounded medical student. We will focus our attention here on gap year students who fall into two other distinct camps: **enhancers** and career **changers**.

Enhancers may have been pre-med in college but struggled to earn good grades or were limited in their extracurricular and volunteering activities that have become "mandatory electives" in the medical school admissions process. The gap years represent a second chance to remediate and improve their application, often in a setting that is more relaxed than the typical pressure-cooker environment of undergraduate pre-med programs.

Career changers are applicants who may have decided to pursue a medical career at the tail end of their undergraduate years or even after graduation and need to fulfill additional requisites to be able to apply to medical school. They may have unique experiences, interests, and achievements in other arenas that will make them competitive in the admissions process, but they need to focus on earning good grades in pre-med classes, getting a respectable score on the MCATs, and gaining clinical exposure if they lack it.

There are many activities that applicants tend to pursue during their gap year(s), depending on what medical school requirements they still need to fulfill (or improve on), and how they can best demonstrate their talents, passions, and altruism in tangible ways. We will discuss each of these in more detail later in the chapter:

- Post-baccalaureate programs
- Special master's programs (SMPs)
- Master's Programs (M.S. or M.A.)
- Extracurricular activities in research and public service
- Hobbies, adventures, and work-related experiences

Applicants who have productive gap years tend to significantly improve the strength of their application. They may have advantages over candidates who applied to medical school during their junior year in college, simply through the additional time in which they were able to bolster their application and cultivate a breadth and depth of experiences, whereas a traditional applicant only has three busy years of college to build her application. In addition to conferring a potentially greater degree of maturity, the extra time off may also demonstrate a level of commitment or perseverance to achieving one's goals. This is looked upon favorably in the admissions process.

While there are clear advantages to taking a gap year or two, the obvious disadvantage is that it delays your career in medicine. Medical school traditionally takes four years and is followed by additional "on the job" training (internship and residency, and for some specialties, fellowship) which can take up to 10 years depending on the specialty you pursue. By delaying medical school, you will be starting your life as a full-fledged physician at a later age. Especially for those applicants for whom debt repayment after medical school is a very real consideration, it is important to think about the amount of income you will lose by taking gap years.

Mend your weaknesses; show your passions

No matter your background, the gap years should be an opportunity for you to improve any major deficits before applying to medical school, as well as to cultivate and deepen your interests.

You may want to use your gap year(s) to fix a low GPA or MCAT score, or maybe you need more time to gather strong letters of recommendation through work, volunteering, or classes. You can also use gap years to explore particular avenues that you may be interested in but have not had the time or fortitude to pursue in the past. These may be not only life-changing and character-building, but will also look good on your application! For instance, if you have an interest in humanitarian work or global health, consider joining the Peace Corps for two years after you graduate from college. If you are interested in underserved communities, apply to teach in an inner-city public school with Teach for America. If you love science and research, consider working as a clinical research coordinator at a medical school, earn a master's degree, or conduct experiments in a laboratory.

Your success will be determined not only by your level of commitment, but also by how wisely you allot your time between résumé-repair versus pursuing interesting extracurricular activities during your gap year(s). Borderline academic applicants who pursue fun activities at the expense of improving their grades and MCAT scores will still find themselves rejected by most schools. Conversely, candidates who ace their pre-baccalaureate coursework but show no humanitarian endeavors or clinical experience will likewise suffer, because they will seem to be one-dimensional.

The worst thing an applicant can do during his or her

gap year is to do nothing at all. This mistake is common among re-applicants, who often live with their parents and do some mundane activities or work, which fails to improve their application. They reapply with the same application the following year, expecting a different outcome—and end up sorely disappointed when they are rejected yet again. Medical schools want applicants who show motivation and intellectual curiosity, taking concrete steps to improve their competitiveness for admission.

In the following sections, we will discuss some common gap-year activities that applicants pursue.

Post-baccalaureate programs

As the name implies, post-baccalaureate programs cater to people who have graduated from college and earned a bachelor's degree. Unlike a graduate program, a post-baccalaureate program does not grant a graduate degree. A pre-medical post-baccalaureate program is popular among pre-med students who are changing careers or looking to improve the below-average GPA they earned throughout college. These programs offer pre-med classes like introductory biology and organic chemistry. Enhancers tend to use these programs to re-take a few classes in which they had previously received a poor grade. Career-changers typically complete their entire set of pre-medical courses within a post-baccalaureate program.

The post-bac program may select instructors and formulate curricula that cater toward pre-med students. For instance, the curriculum may be designed to overlap with the content tested on the MCAT. These programs also offer committee letters, which are comprehensive letters of recommendation amalgamating comments from various professors who have taught in the program and are a good alternative to traditional individual letters of recommendations (see Chapter 6, for more details).

The downside to these programs is that there is greater pressure to perform well. Post-bac programs represent a second chance for applicants to prove they have the academic acumen and study habits necessary to succeed in medical school. Because post-baccalaureate programs are perceived to offer less rigorous courses, it is essential that a student demonstrate his or her ability by earning as high a GPA as possible.

Post-bac programs vary in their cost, quality of instruction, admissions selectivity, student culture, and their relationships with affiliate medical schools, if any. Highly selective post-bac programs typically have fewer seats, stringent admissions criteria, a mission to serve underrepresented students, and may or may not have exclusive linkages with partnered medical schools. A linkage is when a medical school agrees to provisionally accept students from a post-baccalaureate program, provided the student exceeds a certain GPA and MCAT threshold set by the medical school. Less-selective programs are often more expensive, have more seats, have a liberal admissions policy, and rarely if ever have linkage partnerships. Many programs boast their placement statistics, which refer to how many of their graduates end up going to medical school. Be wary of these statistics, as many of them merely reflect what percentage of applicants ended up in any health-related school, including D.O., podiatry, and physical therapy schools.

Regardless of which type of post-baccalaureate program an applicant is enrolled in, it is critical to ace the coursework. Remember, you are competing against other candidates who may be in very similar situation to yours and are just as eager to gain admission to medical school.

Box 8: A career-changer's gap year story

E.K. became interested in global health after he pursued a study abroad semester at the University of Cape Town in South Africa. After breaking his leg in his first game of rugby, he had to go to a local South African hospital and was fascinated by the disparities in healthcare he saw between the poor, local clinics and the posh hospital where he received treatment.

E.K. changed his major from art history to public health during his junior year, with the goal of an academic research career in the field of global health. During the summer of his senior year, he assisted in epidemiological research and did field work on multi-drug resistant tuberculosis in the Tanzanian countryside. It was here that he spent time in many rural clinics and met volunteer physicians from the West who did both clinical practice and research in global health. E.K. realized he enjoyed the hands-on clinical work he observed just as much as he liked academia. He saw those physicians as role models for his envisioned career, and thus transitioned from a PhD route to an MD one.

Over the course of the next two and a half years, E.K. pursued a master's degree in public health while taking additional classes in his spare time, until he fulfilled all his pre-medical course requirements. He then applied to medical schools that had a large focus on global health and offered opportunities for research and stipend-supported fieldwork. He got into the top medical school of his choice and was able to do research and elective rotations in East Africa during school.

If you decide to apply to a post-bac program, you should take the admissions process seriously, as many programs are selective and may vary significantly year-to-year in the number of applications they receive. Make note of whether the program offers all its courses on the same campus, or if its classes are scattered throughout multiple campuses. Also be aware that some programs offer night courses, which may be better for your work schedule.

Do-It-Yourself programs

While post-baccalaureate programs are a good option for some, others opt for a "do-it-yourself" (DIY) route, in which they take classes at a local university but are unaffiliated with any graduate or post-baccalaureate program. If you are currently an undergraduate but plan to take classes after graduating, you may also be able to stay at your university and take a fifth year of classes, depending on your school's policy. The DIY method is especially popular among applicants looking to improve their grades in just a handful of select courses. This method is often more flexible, cheaper, and sidesteps the need to apply for a position within a post-baccalaureate program.

What are the potential downsides? It may be harder to enroll in a given class because enrollment priority may be given to undergraduate students. Post-baccalaureate programs typically reserve and guarantee seats in these classes for their members. Depending on the university, some DIY students also miss out on the post-baccalaureate committee letter. Additionally, an underrated asset of the post-baccalaureate program is how closely knit the students are. Because post-baccalaureate students take the same set of classes at the same time, they form friendships and study partnerships that provide both emotional and scholastic support. In a DIY situation, this kind of network is unlikely to exist because you will be working independently of any program.

Special Master's Programs (SMPs)

These programs are geared toward students who have already taken all of their required pre-med courses and the MCAT but have a non-competitive GPA (roughly below a 3.3). In an SMP, students take advanced graduate-level courses alongside other graduate students and, sometimes, medical students. Students who earn stellar grades in an SMP can demonstrate they can handle the rigor of medical school by performing well in comparable classes that are taken by medical students. This can be a blessing for applicants with low college GPAs, who need to prove they can handle the academic rigors of medical school.

Like post-baccalaureate programs, some SMPs offer

linkages to affiliated medical schools, contingent on exceeding a pre-determined GPA threshold in the SMP. Other programs may guarantee an interview at an affiliated medical school, contingent on satisfactory SMP performance. These programs last 1-2 years and may grant a master's degree upon completion, usually in medical science, biomedical sciences, or health sciences. SMPs vary in their success in getting their students into medical school, with some programs claiming that 80-90% of their students eventually gain admissions to MD or DO medical schools. Note that SMPs also vary in their admissions selectivity, with many programs only admitting around 10-20% of their applicants (so you should apply broadly to maximize your chances of getting into at least one program). Nonetheless, most SMP programs are designed to help applicants with below-average scores and GPAs, so typical SMPs admit students with GPAs ranging from the mid-2.0s to the low-3.0s.

Service-related and research extracurriculars

Many pre-med applicants lack a strong history of volunteering and extracurricular activities during college. To bolster their chances of admission, they often pursue these activities during their gap year. For the borderline applicant, the gap year will be a juggling act of repairing grades, re-taking the MCAT, and fitting in part-time local volunteering. If you fit this profile, we recommend reading the sections on volunteering in Chapter 2.

If your grades, scores, and extracurriculars are already satisfactory, you may want to consider pursuing gap years as a way to immerse yourself in serious extracurricular projects that you either did not have the time for while in college, or may have even already been quite committed to but want to take even further. These activities may revolve around community service, global health, scientific research, athletics, or even a hobby you are passionate about—as long as the activities are serious, sustained, and require an extreme amount of talent or commitment. By pursuing activities that mesh with your interests and goals, you can construct a powerful life story to share in your application essays and interviews. The hallmark of top applicants is their ability to construct and communicate such a cohesive narrative. *For applicants who pursue the most extraordinary paths, the gap year may be what gets you into the top medical schools in the nation.*

If you have a particular interest in research, gap years are an excellent opportunity to focus on that full-time. Many applicants have an interest in clinical research or public health and intend on getting a dual degree at some point in their career. You could choose to earn a master's in that field prior to applying to medical school.

If you need money to make ends meet, consider applying for a full-time research job in a lab.

Box 9: An academic enhancer's gap year story

P.M. majored in biology at her state university and earned a 3.4 GPA. She volunteered at a local free health clinic for three years, eventually becoming a member of the clinic's leadership council and a volunteer trainer. After earning a decent MCAT score, she decided she needed to take a year off to retake a few classes in which she received some C grades.

While retaking several courses at a post-baccalaureate program, P.M. continued her interest in winemaking. While in college, P.M. had taken some classes in the Department of Viticulture and Enology and learned the science of grape growing and winemaking. P.M. worked part time for a large winemaker and ran fermentation analyses. She eventually organized a program with the winemaker that allowed local schoolchildren to see how the grapes are produced and processed into grape juice that is later turned into wine.

P.M. raised her GPA to a 3.65 and applied to medical school. During her interviews, P.M. recalled several times when her interviewers were excited to hear about her highly unusual experiences in winemaking. and the school program she founded.

Many applicants volunteer at a lab and are later hired as paid research assistants. Alternatively, find a job as a clinical research coordinator, where your role will involve assisting with clinical trials and you will have the opportunity to interact directly with patients.

Many applicants may be thinking about a career in global health, and gap years are an excellent opportunity to explore that possibility further. Perhaps the easiest and most widely respected program available is the Peace Corps, which allows American college graduates to live and volunteer in needy parts of the globe to promote education, health, and economic development.

Participants typically serve for two years and receive a living allowance and stipend. Some philanthropic and non-governmental organizations also offer programs that allow college graduates to do research and humanitarian work overseas.

Other candidates are passionate about improving communities at home. If you fall into this category, think about participating in AmeriCorps, Teach for America (TFA), or other similar programs that send educated young people to improve outcomes in the most disadvantaged places in the country. TFA enlists recent college graduates to become teachers in low-income communities for at least two years, while AmeriCorps is a program that mobilizes and coordinates hundreds of volunteer projects across the nation. Some applicants participate in AmeriCorps VISTA, which is like a domestic version of the Peace Corps.

Hobbies and adventures

Many applicants use the gap years as a last 'hurrah' of youth before embarking on their marriage to medicine. While some activities may appear to be the self-indulgent adventures of the well-to-do, many hobbies, jobs, and travels make an applicant stand out from the crowd in a positive way. The possibilities are nearly endless and depend on what your definition of fun is. Many candidates mix pleasure with character-building when they pursue wild adventures and jobs. For instance, an applicant who wants to travel overseas might work as an English instructor in Ecuador while improving his Spanish. Outdoorsy applicants may pursue a job as a wilderness guide, a firefighter, or even a cattle wrangler. Athletic candidates might spend their spare time training for a marathon or an Ironman competition. An accomplished dancer might spend his time living overseas as a dance instructor. Someone with a passion for gardening and sustainable living may consider living and working in a cooperative farming community. In contrast, do not pursue activities that appear selfish, hedonistic, and devoid of character-building or altruism. In other words, do not be the applicant who spends his days windsurfing in a posh Caribbean resort.

While activities like these may make you stand out as a lively and interesting person, it is important to note that they should *not* be a substitute for bad grades, a lack of clinical exposure, or an absence of volunteering experience.

Resources

Here is a list that may help you plan activities to pursue during a gap year:

Unique adventures and jobs:

- EscapeArtist.com

- GapGuru.com

- GapWork.com

- Backdoorjobs.com

- CoolWorks.com

- AdventureJobs.co

Global volunteering, teaching, and working

- PeaceCorps.gov

- GlobalServiceCorps.org

- Careers.amnesty.org

- VolunteerInternational.org

- BUNAC.org

- CIEE.org

- AIESEC.org

Domestic volunteering and public service

- AmeriCorps.gov

- TeachForAmerica.org

- CityYear.org

- Idealist.org

Summary

- Gap years are an increasing trend as applicants look to have more time to build their resumes in an increasingly competitive admissions process. Applicants should weigh the social, emotional, and economic costs of delaying their medical education with the benefits of resume-building during gap years.

- Applicants should balance their time between improving their deficits and developing their side interests.

- Post-baccalaureate programs, DIY programs, and special master's programs are all structured differently and cater toward different needs.

- Gap years can be used for heavy-duty extracurricular activities that can turn a good applicant into a superstar. Pursue activities that are congruent with your interests, goals, and life story

Chapter V

Personal Statement and Secondary Application Essays

O n paper, applicants can appear to be nothing more than an impersonal composite of numbers, facts, and figures, with little to differentiate one individual from another. Really, how can admissions committees tell ten consecutive candidates apart, all highly qualified with GPAs above 3.8 and MCAT scores in the upper echelon? One way is through the personal statement and secondary essays, which are key opportunities for applicants to jump out from the paper and appear dynamic, unique, and—most importantly—human. Besides the interview, these essays represent an applicant's only opportunity to control how they present and package themselves to admissions faculty. Unfortunately, every year, applicants fail to capitalize on this opportunity to present a unique and compelling case for their candidacy. In this chapter, we will discuss how to make your personal statement do much more than the average one—that is to say, how to make it *stand out* from the rest. We will then discuss how to do the same with your secondary essays and cover common prompts. At the end of this chapter, we will include examples of personal statements from applicants who were accepted to medical school.

THE PERSONAL STATEMENT

What is the personal statement?

The personal statement is a 5,300-character essay that all applicants include in their primary application via the American Medical College Application Service (AMCAS). This essay—approximately 1-1.5 pages long when single-spaced—allows applicants to write about the following topics:

- Their suitability for becoming a physician

- Why they want to become a doctor

- Any obstacles they might have encountered in their pre-medical journey

- What vision they have for their future career as a physician

- Any issues or concerns the admissions faculty may have concerning the applicant (e.g., criminal charges, institutional actions, poor grades or scores, time off from school)

This essay requires brainstorming, drafting, and multiple revisions, with the help of friends and mentors as proofreaders. Such a process can require a significant amount of time; therefore, we recommend starting your personal statement several months before submitting it, particularly if you are not a strong or comfortable essay writer. Remember: if you don't complete your personal statement, you cannot submit your application. This delay can then snowball into greater setbacks in later stages of the application process and severely hinder your chances of admission. Since you should be ready to go on the first day applications can be submitted (May 28th in 2020 – typically the last Thursday of May), you should ideally begin working on your statement by February or March of your application year.

How important is the personal statement?

Admissions faculty typically read hundreds personal statements each year. In theory, the personal statement is a vital component of the application process. However, in practice, most applicants write essays that are neither amazingly stirring nor frightfully bad, and therefore do relatively little to affect their chances of admission. As such, the personal statement is —usually – comparatively less critical when compared to other components of the application. In a survey of 142 admissions deans and committee members, personal statements ranked sixth in overall importance, behind science GPA, overall GPA, MCAT scores, letters of recommendation, and clinical volunteering (See Box 2).

That being said, in select instances, a personal statement can make or break a candidate's application. Someone who writes an inspiring, unique, and heartfelt personal statement can stir the emotions of admissions committee members, and this may be the difference between being invited for an interview or not. It may even be the deciding factor that tips the scales in favor of an admit decision. On the other hand, an otherwise strong candidate who submits a sloppy essay rife with spelling errors and questionable content raises a big red flag, which can lead that application file to the "Reject" pile.

What makes a personal statement successful?

To the tired eyes of an admissions committee member,

it can be easy for one personal statement to sound just like the next. Let's face it: it can be challenging to avoid the usual clichés (there are only so many ways to re-phrase the idea that you want to help others, and that you are fascinated by science and the human body) and to figure out how to distinguish your personal state-ment from all the others. In the end, you want to repre-sent yourself accurately and eloquently. While offbeat and quirky essays may capture readers' attentions, if this approach does not really fit your natural style, then you probably don't want to go there.

However, there are other ways to ensure your per-sonal statement works in your favor:

1. It is emotionally resonant

Your reasons for becoming a physician may be large-ly rational or pragmatic, and it's fine to describe these. However, for many applicants, there might have been a particular moment—or sequence of events—that af-fected them deeply and inspired them to enter medi-cine as a profession. If this applies to you, then reflect on a way you can tell your story in an emotionally com-pelling manner that draws your audience in. If you have one entertaining or powerful episode in your life that motivated you to pursue medicine, that may comprise a significant portion of your personal statement. If your decision to enter medicine was gradual and consists of many experiences interspersed over the years, it may be better to give a richly descriptive autobiography of your pre-medical years.

Take advantage of this opportunity to captivate your reader's imagination. Use descriptive language that engages the senses. Do not be afraid to share your feelings or vulnerabilities.

One important point is to make your first paragraph as eye-catching as possible. It is not uncommon for busy admissions members to just skim the rest of the essay if they are bored right from the start. Your introductory sentence, in particular, should grab the attention of your readers and make them want to read on. Some examples of effective opening sentences:

- "In the summer of 2020, I found out first-hand that the lethal dose of a king cobra's venom is about 200 milligrams."

- "By the end of the night, there were nearly 30,000 soles aboard the ship—shoe soles, that is."

- "In my 26th straight hour of guarding the cattle, I discovered there is such a thing as not only a second wind, but also a third, and a fourth."

At the same time, you must temper an eye-popping style and avoid any possibility that you will offend your reader through your subject matter and/or language. Steer clear from topics that are likely to offend a large proportion of admissions officers. Topics like abortion, birth control, politics, and religion should generally be avoided, unless they represent the cornerstone of your application (for example, if you run an organization that distributes contraceptives to an underserved community). Refrain from bold statements that seem too self-congratulatory, naive, or melodramatic (e.g., "I was the only one in my community strong enough to succeed"; "Going from being a child who had a mother with cancer to an oncogene researcher, I am now one step closer to finding the cure for cancer and making my mom proud.")

---

2. It paints a cohesive narrative in which your extracurricular activities fit together and make sense

For too many applicants, the personal statement is simply a bland recitation of each extracurricular activity they completed as a pre-med student.

> **Box 10: Should your personal statements address your weak points?**
>
> Admissions officers may raise an eyebrow when they review an applicant with a low GPA, a low MCAT score, multiple class withdrawals, or an institutional action (e.g., academic probation, possession of alcohol in the college dormitory). It is no surprise some applicants wonder whether they should proactively address these weak points in their personal statement.
>
> While it may seem appropriate to acknowledge and explain any red flags in your application in the context of your personal statement, we recommend you focus on your strong points instead. If you devote your essay to "damage control," even if you describe how you have become a stronger and better person as a result, the reader ends up thinking of you in that specific context more so than according to your strengths ("Oh, that's the applicant who was caught up in that cheating scandal during his freshman year.") Use your essay to show who you are at your best. There are other, more appropriate ways to address your weak points (e.g., your interview and secondary essays).

The essay merely jams these together like cramming two puzzle pieces together that don't fit, with the end result being a disjointed mess. How and why, for instance, did you go from working as a physical trainer to a hospice care volunteer, and then from there to a clinical researcher on muscular dystrophy? Your essay should outline how experience X shaped your character and motivations, and how this personal change led to your decision to pursue experience Y, and then how Y led to Z, and so on. Rather than describe in detail what you did in each activity, focus on how these activities made you grow as a person and developed your motivation to become a doctor. If you have a hard time coming up with enough relevant experiences, this may be a sign your resume is a bit too thin, and you should consider pursuing more activities before applying to medical school.

While writing this narrative, be sure you tackle the main purpose of the personal statement, which is why you want to be a doctor. Review Chapter 1 for the most common good and bad reasons many applicants decide to pursue medicine.

---

3. It is polished and has the right tone

All too often, we read personal statements that are disorganized, incoherent, or full of spelling and grammatical errors. The essay may also come across as overly conversational (e.g., full of slang and contractions) or, conversely, too pretentious (e.g., florid language or complicated syntax). Do NOT use expletives or profane language, even if you think it works well within the context of what you are writing about (you never know whether such language may offend the particular admissions committee member reading your essay). These kinds of mistakes are easily avoidable, yet they make their way into applicants' personal statements every year in shockingly high numbers. If an applicant makes such careless mistakes in such an important essay, it does not reflect well on his or her character. The candidate appears to be sloppy, clueless, or apathetic—all of which are terrible qualities to have in a future physician.

SECONDARY ESSAYS

What are secondary essays?

After submitting your primary application—which includes your personal statement—medical schools review your application and may send you a *secondary* application. For most schools, the secondary application includes requests for one or more secondary essays that you are required to complete, with the recommended length typically limited to 200-1,000 words per essay. While the essay prompts (topics) differ from one school to the next, there are several common themes that frequently come up time and again.

The purpose and importance of the secondary essay

Like the personal statement, the purpose of secondary essays is for the admissions committee to learn even more about you who are as a person, including your life experiences, values, personal characteristics, and aspirations. They are used by medical schools to determine whether you are a good fit for the values and emphases of their program in particular. For instance, a medical school focused on primary care and rural medicine may prompt applicants to write about their experiences with the underserved. Top medical schools focus on scientific research and leadership, and so they often ask their applicants to explain their pre-med research and leadership experiences in depth.

Therefore, when completing these secondary essays, keep in mind each school's particular philosophy and values.

Research the mission statement of the school; some school websites even state, specifically, what kind of students they are seeking.

Secondary essay strategies

Clearly, given that each school has different admissions selection criteria and priorities, a *customized* approach is necessary for filling out your secondary essays as you explain why you are a good fit for that individual school. It is not necessary to repeat what you have already covered in your personal statement in the primary application, unless there is a particular element or activity worth embellishing upon because you were limited by space constraints originally.

Many secondary essay prompts are open-ended, offbeat, or even somewhat unusual, and give applicants wide latitude to respond however they like. These may be included to get a better sense of an applicant's creative side or personality, and you should feel free to use this opportunity to show the unique side of yourself. At the same time, you should still respond in a way that highlights to the admissions committee such laudable qualities and experiences as humility, altruism, overcoming challenges, contributing diversity to the medical institution, and leadership.

You should aim to complete your secondary essays within two weeks of receiving your secondary application, as many schools have a short turnaround deadline and view late submissions unfavorably. If you are applying to a large number of schools (30+), you may even want to consider writing some of these essays *before* receiving your secondary application. However, if you opt to go with this strategy, you will need to search for the essay questions elsewhere, such as the Student Doctor Network online discussion forums at http://forums.studentdoctor.net.

What follows are some common secondary essay prompts and how you might choose to respond. Note that these prompts are often used as interview questions, too.

Most common prompts

---

1. 'What have you been doing since applying?"

Obviously, it does not look particularly good if you

have stopped most of the extracurricular activities you pursued before applying to medical school...so don't. This gives the impression that your interests and altruism were merely a show for the admissions committee. Even better than merely continuing your primary interests while applying to medical school, ideally you are taking on greater leadership roles within the organizations of which you are a part of. Show you are serious about, and committed to, your future career path by emphasizing your volunteering efforts, community service helping those that are marginalized or vulnerable, and patient-centric work. Research-heavy schools may like to hear about progress you've made in whatever research project you've been involved in, including new publications and presentations.

---

2. 'Describe the most challenging (or rewarding) experience in your life."

This is a nice opportunity for you to share something particularly meaningful to you, and in the process, highlight some personal qualities that show why you will be a good physician in the future. For some applicants, answering this question may be easy: for instance, if you were first to graduate college in your extended family, you can mention graduating as your most challenging or rewarding experience, then discuss the obstacles it took to get there which demonstrate traits of perseverance and an appealing trailblazing sort of nature.

On the other hand, if you come from a more privileged background, it may be useful to reflect on a time you helped another person and why it was particularly rewarding. While it may be true that completing your first marathon was challenging and showed qualities of self-discipline and dedication, applicants who choose to write about their service to others—rather than about themselves—are generally more well-received as it shows a more altruistic, outward-looking focus. One possible exception to this is if you are applying to a medical school that greatly values research, in which case it might be reasonable to talk about a particularly difficult time taking charge of a research project and how you overcame those difficulties to produce presentable scientific work.

---

3. 'Discuss how your life experiences have contributed to prevailing over adversity or have enhanced your ability to add diversity to our community."

If you are an underrepresented minority or have ever been socioeconomically disadvantaged, this is a prime opportunity to discuss that at length. If you have any interest in treating the underserved as a physician, make special note of this. For applicants who do not personally fit this mold, focus on any community service that enhanced your exposure to diverse populations. For instance, if you worked with a health clinic that primarily served persons of color, you can mention that fact and how it improved your cultural awareness and competence.

Acknowledging that not all applicants may have worked with disenfranchised or minority populations, the term "diversity" can be open to some degree of interpretation. You may have a talent or hobby that adds to the diversity of the student body. Schools love applicants who are serious athletes, artists, or multilingual. Any unique or quirky hobbies can also be described here, for instance, being a cake decorator, a wine maker, or a semi-professional curler.

---

4. 'Why do you want to attend our school?"

The real answer might be "I don't unless I have to— you're my back-up school" or "I just get excited thinking about the name of your school," but secondary essays require a more diplomatic response.

Oftentimes, your answer to this prompt can be a critical determinant of whether you are invited to an interview or not. If you are a highly qualified candidate, less selective schools may be skeptical of whether you will actually matriculate because they anticipate you will receive offers from higher-ranked schools. Elite, highly selective schools want to know you are applying for specific reasons and not just because they're in the U.S. News and World Report's Top Ten list.

If you dig deep enough, you can find something you would like about any medical school in the United States. This could be its location, curriculum, faculty, cost, affiliated hospitals, its mission and values, the patient population, or its emphases (e.g., global health, translational research, local community outreach). For each school with this prompt, you should research all of these aspects and make note of the ones that are of greatest value to you. Bring up your past experiences and activities as proof of your interest in whatever you like about the school. Be specific and give details whenever possible, to demonstrate you have substantive reasons for wanting to attend that school.

An example would be an applicant interested in the Yale School of Medicine. Yale has many strengths, including global health, basic science research, and translational/clinical research. An applicant with no overseas experiences or any personal connection to Connecticut might sound disingenuous detailing how he or she is enamored of Yale's global health programs or that they have always wanted to live in New Haven. If he or she has experience and interest in clinical research, however, then their essay could focus on how they would love the opportunity to pursue this at Yale. The more specific, the better.

Using this case as an illustration, here is an example of a mediocre response:

I have participated in scientific research while in college and have come to love it. The reason I want to go to Yale is that it has a strong reputation for research. At Yale, I would continue to do research to strengthen my skills as a physician-investigator, and then pursue research later in my career. Yale offers a number of research programs that I would like to be involved in, especially regarding neuroscience.

Much better would be the following:

My experiences volunteering at an Alzheimer's care center helped me notice some of the perceptual deficits many patients had. This piqued my curiosity and I investigated how an Alzheimer's drug affects plasticity in the occipital lobe of the brain. I hope to go to Yale to continue the same approach, in which everyday observations shape the kind of research I do. Yale has a marvelous system to promote this style of inquiry, with its academic advisor program, thesis program, and the fifth-year option, which I would take to hone and develop my research into substantive work. I am interested in programs like YCCI and VBT, which are proof of Yale's commitment to working with a diverse set of professionals to bridge the gap between bench and bedside.

This paints a more vibrant picture of the student's research interests and experience, and by describing specific aspects of Yale's medical training programs that attract her, she shows that she has done her homework and is applying for reasons beyond the superficial.

---

5. 'Discuss any additional information you would like to bring to the attention of the admissions committee."

Here might be the right opportunity to address any glaring red flags in your application file. If you have an institutional action, criminal charges, a semester of particularly bad grades, or some other weak spot, you should explain the circumstances surrounding why you made the mistake, how you have learned and grown from it, and how you have taken all the necessary steps to correct it. If none of these apply to you, then of course you have room to further accentuate and expound upon any positives in your application that you did not have room to discuss in detail previously. This might involve an interesting tidbit about your family or upbringing, another activity you were involved in that meant a lot to you, or some aspect of your personality or character that you think bears emphasizing.

Less common questions

1. 'Are there any gaps in your education? Explain."

This refers to any time you took off in between college and applying to medical school (i.e., "gap years"), or extended time-off during your college years. If you decided to change careers and pursue a career in medicine only after you graduated from college, explain your reasons for doing so. If you needed to take time off to help during a major family illness or financial crisis or had to make money for a period so that you could even afford medical school, it is fine to mention these as well. Try to describe what you were doing as productive and meaningful. If you took a year off to travel the world, explain how this afforded you first-hand and up-close cross-cultural experiences, rather than just allowed you to have fun and take a break from studies.

2. 'How do you envision your career in the future?"

Keep in mind that admissions committees recognize that a candidate's initial vision of what their career looks like prior to entering medical school may evolve over the next four years, shaped in part by what they're exposed to during these formative years of training...and that such change is entirely fine, and expected. So, in some ways, there is no "wrong" answer to this question (unless you envision a cushy 9-to-5 job with high pay and low stress)...and no one is holding you to your answer or keeping track after the fact. So simply be honest here—it's OK even to be somewhat idealistic, as long as you don't come across seeming naïve and uninformed. Acknowledge if you don't know with absolute certainty what your career will look like, but provide at least some of your initial thoughts or ideas. Also use the opportunity to explain why the school to which you are applying will help you to pursue these future career goals. For instance, if you envision a career studying tropical disease, you can mention how the school's global health partnerships in equatorial Africa would allow you to volunteer during your medical school summers in regions where tropical diseases are endemic. You should generally explain how your career goals are informed by your current passions, and how you have pursued these interests in the past.

---

3. 'Give an autobiography, including your family, childhood, school years, and what you have done after college, if applicable. Explain what led you to pursue medicine during this life story."

Most schools that use this question give a 1.5-2 page limit, making it one of the longest secondary essays you are likely to write. For most schools that ask this prompt, it will be the only secondary essay you write. The hardest part of writing this essay will be to not repeat your personal statement, which may resemble an autobiography. This prompt is somewhat open-ended, analogous to the common interview question of, "Tell me about yourself." A clear chronological narrative with a logical story arc of your path toward medicine is the most straightforward, but not necessarily the only way to answer this prompt. You can, for example, use a powerful and seminal moment from any point in your life as a starting point, and then work backward and forward from there. A funny anecdote or poignant story can help break up the recitative nature of the essay. Feel free to be a little creative if you are a particularly good writer.

---

4. 'Describe your research project(s) in detail, including hypothesis, results, and analysis."

An important rule of thumb: be able to explain your research, whether on paper or in person, in a way that the average person can understand. Avoid technical jargon and scientific minutiae as much as you can. Explain why the work is important and (if applicable) how it may ultimately benefit patients. If possible, give a draft to your research mentor so he or she can lend their expertise and ensure your essay is accurate and readable.

Unusual prompts that you might encounter

1. "Discuss your weaknesses and how you plan on improving them."

2. "What do you think will be your greatest challenges in medical school?"

3. "Discuss a time you received negative feedback or were in a confrontational situation. How did you react?"

4. "What was your most humbling experience and why?"

Summary

- The personal statement is a required component of your primary application. It should focus on why you want to be a doctor and, if applicable, any major obstacles you have faced. Your reasons should be grounded in experience.

- Drafting a personal statement requires multiple revisions and proofreaders. This takes time; don't make the mistake of taking too long to start and finalize your personal statement.
  An exceptionally good or bad personal statement can affect your odds of admission, but the vast majority tend to have relatively minimal impact on an applicant's chances.

- Start your personal statement in a way that will grab the reader's attention. An emotionally resonant story, a clear narrative of how you arrived at this current point in your career, and clean writing are all worthwhile goals in your essay.

- Secondary essays are often important for securing an interview and are largely used to determine whether an applicant is a good fit for the school's institutional values and mission. You should offer your activities and experiences as demonstrable evidence that you possess universally valued characteristics such as leadership, resilience, and altruism.

- Secondary essays are also good practice for interviews because the essay prompts resemble common interview questions.

Successful Personal Statements

Example 1:

Everyone has moments of self-doubt. In 2008, I had recently graduated from B University and was working as a teaching assistant in biology. Things were coming together and it seemed like my goal of becoming the first doctor in our family was actually achievable. A lot of hard work remained, but by then, I had overcome many obstacles and none of the remaining ones seemed insurmountable. It was then, on an otherwise ordinary Sunday when I was preparing my teaching plan for the following week that I received a distraught phone call from my estranged biological father to watch the evening news. A young male was gunned down during a police standoff. It was my older brother, J. I felt a torrent of emotions. My brother who was my best friend and emotional rock was taken from me and I was left feeling empty. His sudden passing brought self-doubt to the surface and made me remember where I came from and wonder why I wanted to pursue medicine.

J was the main positive male role model in my life. Both my biological father and my stepfather were not around consistently and although J did not live with me, we always kept in touch. He was the one who encouraged me not to give up when things at home became financially challenging. He was the one who comforted me when I got bullied at school for being different. He was the one who helped inspired me towards medicine. Sharing a single room with my mother, my unreliable stepfather, and my younger brother, we made the best of our situation. The tipping point came when I started high school and my parents separated. My mother took on more work to support us and I was forced to help fill in the gaps. J reassured me that things would get better. He made sure that I did not fall behind in my studies when I had to take on a part-time job.

School, unfortunately, was not a refuge from the stress at home. With a mixed Filipino and African-American heritage, my classmates who did not understand why I looked and acted differently harassed me. J would listen patiently as I shared with him my feelings of isolation and identity. He gave me advice that at the time I did not fully understand. He told me not to let those kids bring me down because I was special. "You are different for a reason; you are able to navigate both of your parents' cultures and will have a unique understanding of other people and the world." This unique understanding was soon tested when I suggested that my younger brother receive medical treatment for

his escalating symptoms of bipolar disorder. To my mother, it was perceived as an act of betrayal as we did not discuss family matters to outsiders. All I wanted to do was to protect my little brother. J told me not to blame myself and to focus on the things I could do for him. In my limited capacity, I set out to learn all I could about his illness and became the link between his doctors and my mother. By helping to bridge the cultural divide, I was able to provide comfort to her and allow my brother to get treatment. This was my first push towards medicine. I saw how such an earth shattering family event was met by doctors who were willing and able to piece our family back together again. I was inspired by their breadth of science and by the compassion in which they approached our situation. J was very proud of how I handled the crisis. He suggested that I should become a doctor. Growing up, I never imagined going to college, let alone attending medical school, as I had to often push my own personal goals aside for my family's survival. But if J believed in me, then I knew I could do it. With his encouragement and my own motivation to help others, I worked diligently and earned a scholarship to B University.

J's tragic death, however, called everything into question and brought a sense of insecurity to the surface. Could I do it without him and find the strength to move ahead? He always helped me navigate through the obstacles I faced and now I turned inwards to find my own compass to guide me back to medicine. I took time off to find the answer for myself over the next few years. Immersing myself in medicine as a research coordinator I found a new source of inspiration. I was presented with an elderly Chinese immigrant man suffering from heart failure who had no local family. For me, family meant everything - support, encouragement, guidance. I empathized with how difficult his condition would be to face alone. Thus, I stepped up to walk him through the process as he received a pacemaker that transformed his life. Working closely with him, I rediscovered my passion that pushed me towards medicine in the first place - to help patients both physically and emotionally. I realized that even though J is no longer with me, the lessons he taught me and the ones that I have acquired through my clinical experiences will propel me forward and help me succeed as a physician. I know that there will be days and situations that will seem overwhelming, but I have learned to see the potential in myself and in others, and together with the people I will care for, I will work hard to help them thrive.

This student attended a top 10 ranked medical school.

Example 2:

"Step. Step. Rock step." When I was a boy, my grandmother and I would say those words together. It helped us when we danced. Nothing made her happier, and dancing helped to spark old memories. When she was diagnosed with Alzheimer's disease, dancing became our way of connecting to each other and to her past. Toward the end, it was our only way to connect.

How could she still remember how to dance, but yet she could not remember what she had eaten that morning? How could the simple act of dancing cause her to become more lucid? Why did she still have her older memories, and why were they more active when danced? These questions had a scientific explanation, and, at the same time, were very personal. These ruminations also sparked an interest in medicine for me.

In college, I learned there are different kinds of memory: episodic, semantic, working, and procedural. I remembered how my grandmother's ailment diminished each aspect, until only her procedural memory persisted. The automatic skills we acquire—like riding a bike, playing the piano, or reading—can be the most enduring. When we danced, I realized it was a ritual through which she could express her character despite her illness.

The more I learned, the more I wanted to investigate

the science behind our behaviors and experiences. I began to assist in research at H College. I took an interest in not only how the brain works, but how it affects clinical populations. It was not enough to investigate how a system worked. I had to know how that knowledge could be applied when those systems go awry. It was not enough to know how a certain neurotransmitter modulated a certain part of the brain. I had to know how that affected a patient's behavior, or how that information could be adapted to design a new drug.

New questions sprang to mind. They seemed more exciting if they had clinical ramifications. For example: Why is it that 90 percent of people with schizophrenia are heavy smokers? Why would a certain enzyme inhibitor be helpful to people with Alzheimer's disease? While doing laboratory research on these two questions, I felt invigorated. I had always loved science, and now I was getting to apply it in an effective way. I found an interesting answer to the first question: Perhaps they smoke because the nicotine can be shown to improve their perceptual cognitive deficits. This possibility got me fascinated in psychopharmacology and perceptual learning, which investigates how drugs affect procedural memory. I conducted a study on Aricept, which is an Alzheimer's drug that affects acetylcholine levels in the brain. My findings are now being prepared for journal publication.

While doing research, I met and read about physicians who not only practice medicine but also do research. I began to consider the possibility of being more than an academic. To that end, I began to volunteer in clinical settings. I found that I enjoyed being with patients, and that being with them only enriched my experiences as a researcher.

Every week I spend time with people with Alzheimer's disease, and they have fostered in me a greater sense of compassion. We've established close bonds and they share their most abiding memories which have yet to vanish. One woman often recalls, "My father took care of us when my mother died. He was a cook, and he loved us." Another always says, "When I was younger I travelled the world. I've never wanted to stay in one place."

As I came to appreciate the patients around me, serving them became a rich and gratifying experience.

While volunteering, I noticed how often a sickness robs someone of their dignity. A hospital patient cannot speak because her mouth is full of fluid and she can't expectorate. Another one feels powerless because he cannot remember the place where he proposed to his wife. In cases like these, I remember being able to help patients in whatever small way I could, and they expressed a measure of gratitude that made me feel whole. I saw nurses and physicians around me providing their expert care, and I marveled at how they applied their training toward the same end but to an even greater effect.

During a vacation, I traveled with a friend to a town on the East African coast. We spent four weeks shadowing physicians at a public hospital and many of its departments. I saw patients questioned, wounds stitched, suprapubic catheters inserted, and a number of other procedures. The sheer variety and complexity of the procedures made me more interested in medicine beyond the scope of the brain. I also became acutely aware of how a hospital's procedures, policies, and resources are directly tied to patient health outcomes.

After observing health care professionals in clinical and research settings, I came to realize that I want to follow their example. There is something magical about combining scientific knowledge, research, keen observation, inquisitiveness, and patient-centered care to save and improve lives. There is a deep sense of reward that comes with alleviating pain and restoring dignity to someone in need. With all these things in mind, I know without a doubt that I want to be a physician.

This student attended a top 10 ranked medical school.

Example 3:

My dream was to become a professional soccer player. I scrutinized and mastered my favorite players' signature moves, down to the angles of their shots. I often trained alone until the field lights turned off, hours after my teammates went home. Naturally, when my club soccer coach appointed me as team captain, my ten-year-old self was elated and proud. I naively flaunted the "captain" band around my arm, trying to lead with the loudest voice and the most talent. However, over the years, I learned that leading a team requires greater responsibility and attentiveness to each teammate's talents and contributions.

When I tore my ACL in high school, I was hopeless and heartbroken. The pain of jeopardizing my soccer career was equal to, if not greater than, the physical pain in my knee. However, I remember my orthopedic surgeon, Dr. D, taking the time and care to walk me through the treatment process step-by-step during this time of vulnerability. As we looked at the MRI and monitored the stages of my recovery, I was intrigued by the restorative power of the body. He showed me the anatomy of my torn ACL and explained the mechanisms that my body used to heal itself. During my year-long treatment, I was always eager to meet Dr. D to learn more about the progress of my knee and how to properly rehabilitate it. In the months of reflection during my recovery, my ego-fueled pursuit of becoming a soccer player was challenged by my insight into our fragility and necessity for medicine.

Throughout college, the passion and devotion I once had for soccer shifted towards an interest in learning more about medicine. I wanted to participate in caring for the underserved, so I joined Community Restoration (CR) medical clinic. There, I worked with multiple physicians as they provided free health care to the homeless in the city. Over the years, I became close to C, a home-less woman who regularly came to our clinic. She walked in each time with a fresh and gaping wound on her arm; however, the physician and I had trouble diagnosing the problem because she would not tell us the cause of the injury. Nevertheless, the provider taught me how to treat the wounds, and I tended to her each time. After building a friendship with C, she opened up to me and shared that she inflicted the wounds on herself just to be seen and treated by a doctor. I soon realized she simply yearned the love and care that she did not receive on the streets. As C's tears dripped onto my shoulder, I realized that the homeless people I was serving deserved just as much love and care as any of us. If anything, they need extra care and attention due to their circumstances. Through C and serving the homeless, I learned that a physician has the duty and opportunity to not only heal physically, but also to heal emotionally.

After volunteering at CR, I hungered to learn even more about medicine, so I applied to be a medical scribe for L Hospital. After observing doctors on the hospital floor, I saw how gracefully each physician juggled diagnosing patient's problems, directing residents and nurses, and making important decisions in high-stress environments. They led the medical team and utilized the strengths of each nurse, scribe, and technician to ultimately better the health of each patient. I noticed that the physicians led in a way that fostered an environment in which each member of the medical team had a voice and felt like a contributor to the team. As a scribe, I saw the parallel between the leadership of a physician and that of a soccer team captain. Moreover, I recognized that leadership as a physician had deeper meaning, as its purpose is not to win matches and gain personal satisfaction but to heal the sick and make a lasting impact on the community. Beyond leadership, I admired that physicians are always mentoring and learning, especially in academic medicine. I observed doctors send labs to one another, collaborate on innovative techniques, and discuss rare cases as part of their daily work. Working as a scribe for two years, I witnessed how the role of a physician extends beyond treating the patient, but includes working harmoniously with colleagues to provide the best health care possible.

Though my treatment process with Dr. D is what initially attracted me to becoming a doctor, my time at CR and L Hospital cemented my desire to pursue it as a career. These experiences, though varied, demonstrated how medicine was the perfect culmination of my three biggest passions: learning, serving, and collaborating. I am looking forward to learn constantly as a physician-scientist about the intricacies and restorative nature of the body. Additionally, I wish to continue to work with the underserved population to physically and emotionally heal patients like C. Finally, I strive not to be the flaunting "captain" that I once was for my soccer team, but to be a physician leader that emphasizes teamwork and humility.

As my dream has changed from being a professional soccer player to a doctor, I aim to relentlessly train to become a physician leader that can make an impact on individual patients and the community as a whole.

This student attended a top 20 ranked medical school.

Example 4:

"I don't know if I can do this alone," J whispered. I felt helpless processing her words, but I listened to my instinct and knelt to look into her eyes. Beneath the fluorescent lights of the exam room, she confided in me her story of hiding a part of her identity for most of her life–the isolation, the piercing stares and whispers that followed when she came out as transgender, and her dream of dancing on stage when she no longer feels the need to hide her body. The years of waiting were over; the day of her gender affirmation surgery was here. As she grasped my hands in hers, I realized what she needed most in this moment was to feel heard and supported. The concept of individualized care was no longer abstract. Looking into J's eyes, I had a newfound respect for its true gravity. Medicine is the field in which I can forge impactful relationships informed by my understanding of patients' cultures and experiences.

My journey to helping patients like J began at the

City Free Clinic (CFC) when I met C, a patient who spoke passionately about the dignified care he received there. Every shift, I looked forward to seeing C's gentle smile as he told me about everything from his bike rides to the latest book he read at the library. One day, however, I found him in a state of distress. His eyes filled with tears as he angrily screamed that his bike and sleeping bag had been stolen, and along with them, his feeling of security. My colleague suggested we initiate a psychiatric hold, but I recalled the traumatic experiences C had shared with me and offered to talk to him privately first. As I reassured him I would not leave until he felt safe, his trembling slowly ceased. I helped him call mental health resources and promised to check on him the following week. The trust we had built allowed me to support him in a vulnerable moment. My relationship with C will always serve as a reminder of how powerful human connection is, and showed me I want a profession in which I can connect with people and help them during their most difficult times. Through a career in medicine, I hope to create sincere, longitudinal relationships in order to care for an individual's intimate health needs.

While volunteering at the CFC, a patient introduced me to Dr. B's work for the transgender community. "She is a genius, an artist, and an advocate," the patient said, convincing me I wanted to learn from this physician. During my first week of volunteering for her, Dr. B walked me through her surgery plan with a clear vision and focus. As she explained that the goal of the surgery is to reverse a patient's current anatomy to their prenatal configuration, she emphasized the complexity of achieving a result that is not only functional but also aesthetic. She shared, "No two bodies are the same," and that she must constantly adapt her surgery plan to the goals of each patient. I noticed how Dr. B was able to use her clinical knowledge to help patients feel complete in their identity. I craved the ability to comprehend patients' backgrounds informed by medical understanding in this way. Dr. B encouraged me to reach out to patients and understand their stories.

That is how I found myself in the exam room with J. I observed Dr. B greet J by her preferred name, beginning by asking about her life and transition experience. "Working with this community for over 15 years has taught me how much more you learn about a patient through their story rather than seeing them as just a medical history," Dr. B later shared. Dr. B asked J about her love for dance in an effort to create a comfortable environment. J then revealed that she felt anxious about surgical complications. Dr. B reassured J that while she could not promise things would go perfectly, she would be by her side every step of the way. Because of her cultural understanding and expertise in transgender health, Dr. B guided J through this life-changing experience in a way nobody else could. After her surgery, J hugged Dr. B. "I will always remember today as the day my life began," J said. In this moment, I was humbled by the privilege physicians have to build such rare, profound relationships with their patients. Although I will not share the lived experiences of every patient, I hope to become a physician who immerses themselves in the culture and experiences of their patients.

I have witnessed patients' lives being inextricably intertwined with those who provide their care. People can overcome remarkable challenges when their health is cared for by someone they trust. C became a volunteer and has since empowered countless others through his lived experience. J auditioned for her university's dance team and has performed in front of thousands of people. Medicine is an integration of the science of healing and careful regard for patients' individual needs. When patients present in unideal, vulnerable situations, physicians have the unique responsibility to connect with them and improve their health in a lasting way. My desire to build patient relationships grounded in trust and devotion to understanding patients' experiences motivate me to pursue a career in medicine.

Chapter VI

Letters of Recommendation

The challenge of admissions is figuring out who an applicant truly is beyond their collection of scores and grades. Some of this can come from the personal statement and other essays, as well as personal interviews if the candidate is lucky enough to be invited. But another absolutely essential component are the letters of recommendation. These letters provide an opportunity for admissions committees to get a much clearer sense of what professors, work or laboratory supervisors, and/or other respected figures of authority really think of a given applicant: Are they all that they profess to be in their application file? Are they a superstar or just a solid, above-average student? Are they truly passionate about caring for the underserved, or do they show up to the homeless clinic every few weeks? In one survey (see Box 18), letters of recommendation were only second to interview performance in deciding which interviewees to accept—and were more important than MCAT scores and GPAs.

The reality is that there is significant variability in the quality of letters we review during the admissions process. Sometimes, these letters represent the pivot point for why an applicant is ultimately rejected or accepted. To get truly outstanding letters, you must have the right strategy. That means knowing whom to ask, when to ask, how to ask, and how many to ask for a letter of recommendation. We will also cover what makes a good letter versus a mediocre one, and how you can receive the best letters possible.

How do letters of recommendation work?

There are two main kinds of letters of recommendation: individual letters and committee letters. Students may choose to acquire a collection of letters from mentors, supervisors, professors, physicians, and more. These letter writers independently submit their letters to the medical schools to which the student applied. Conversely, most post-baccalaureate pre-medical programs, as well as some undergraduate schools, instead opt to send out a committee letter on behalf of its students, either in lieu of or in addition to individual letters. This letter is written by a pre-medical advising committee also require students to fill out a questionnaire or meet with them in person to get a better sense of their background, activities, goals, and personality. The committee then aggregates and synthesizes the information to do one of two things: (1) generate a comprehensive letter highlighting all of the applicant's accomplishments and strengths, with long excerpts from the individual letter-writers embedded within; or (2) form the individual letters (kept verbatim and in full) into a packet with a cover letter attached (which is typically much shorter than the full-length letter in #1).

Of note, unlike the old days, a letter-writer rarely can simply mail his letter of recommendation to the medical schools to which the candidate has applied. First, the letter must pass through a letter-forwarding service. These services are holding tanks that collect letters of recommendation for an applicant and then send those letters out to the medical schools when the applicant wishes to do so. The advantage of this service is that the letter writer only needs to send the letter to one destination—the letter forwarding service—rather than separately to each of the 20 or 30 or more medical schools to which the candidate may have applied. However, there are a number of letter-forwarding services available, and it is important to realize that the relationship between letter writers, forwarding services, and medical schools can be labyrinthine.

There are three main letter-forwarding services: Interfolio, VirtualEvals, and AMCAS, all of which are free of charge. Additionally, if your school or post-bac pro-gram uses a committee letter, check to make sure they will take care of the letter forwarding on your behalf, which is typically the case. Any of these services will forward your letters to all the American MD schools to which you apply. (Note that VirtualEvals and Interfolio usually just send these letters onto AMCAS, from which medical schools can then directly download their appli-cants' letters of recommendations.)

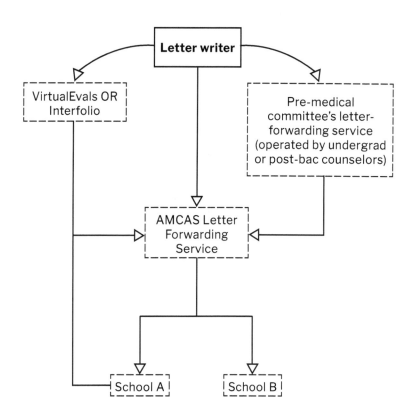

Of note, applicants can apply to medical schools without having all of their letters of recommendation submitted. However, the vast majority of schools will not consider inviting someone to interview unless they submit the minimum number of required letters of recommendation. This often ends up being the reason why applicants who otherwise submitted their application materials early end up falling behind during interview season—unfair, perhaps, but all the more reason to make sure you are on top of getting your letter-writers to submit their letter on your behalf in a timely fashion!

Because AMCAS only holds onto letters for one year, it may be useful to use another letter-forwarding service that holds letters for a longer period. We will discuss this more in the section titled "When to ask".

Letter confidentiality

Applicants have the right to read a letter of recommendation before submitting it—but they also have the option to waive that right. The applicant's decision is made known to the letter writer and to the medical schools reviewing the letters.

To waive or not to waive? This may seem like one of the biggest dilemmas an applicant can face, although it is important to keep in mind that many busy letter-writers simply never check to see whether an applicant has waived his letters of recommendation or not. That being said, there may be occasional professors who will not agree to write a letter of recommendation if they know you will be able to read it, as they may feel this hampers their ability to speak freely and honestly. Additionally, as a general principle, medical schools tend to prefer confidential letters because they are perceived as more candid and less likely to be cherry-picked by the applicant. After all, an applicant who reads his own letters can readily submit only the good ones and conveniently toss out the ones that are less than sterling—and where is the objectivity in that?

Box 11: How to make sure your letters are good without breaking author confidentiality

One problem is that no matter how strong you think a letter is going to be, you really cannot be sure. But you don't have to read the letter yourself (and waive its confidentiality) in order to be certain of its quality.

If you have a pre-med committee that writes committee letters, you can forward your letters to the committee. You can ask your counselors at the committee to read your letters and inform you if any are less than laudatory. If they are, you have the right to request that they not be included in your submission.

If you do not have the luxury of a committee, one common, and effective, tactic is to ask each of your letter writers if they can write you a strong letter. Ask them to be honest with you. If they cannot, hopefully they will be forthright about it or gently suggest that you might be better off looking elsewhere for a letter. Many students may feel it is awkward to ask so blunt a question—and it is—but a few moments of discomfort can help ensure that this core component of your application is as bulletproof as it can be.

What is the main advantage to *not* waiving your right to see your letters? Primarily this: a bad, or even mediocre letter of recommendation can seriously damage an applicant's chances of admission, especially when competing against other candidates who have uniformly glowing letters touting them as the best thing since sliced bread. If you are not sure how your professor really feels about you (did he notice those couple of times you skipped lecture?), or how well he really knows you, it may behoove you *not* to waive your right to see your letter. Alternatively, there are other methods to ensure all the letters you send out are highly favorable, while still waiving your right to see them, as described in Box 11.

How many letters should I get?

Applicants often assume that the more letters they include, the better, the same way a Hollywood starlet might measure her reputation by the number of fan letters she receives. The problem with that reasoning is that including any letters that are mediocre may actually *detract* from your application. The best strategy is to focus on quality over quantity: only include the letters you think are likely to be very strong and, ideally, as personal as possible. These letters should paint an intimate portrait of you that highlights your strongest attributes while minimizing any negatives (let alone fatal flaws). If your letters are a mixed bag of bad and good opinions, then medical schools will think you're a mixed bag, too.

The caveat, of course, is that you *must* get a minimum number of letters. Many schools impose their own letter requirements, which you will have to research before applying to each school. Some of these schools have categorical requirements, meaning, for example, at least one letter from a science professor whose course you took. The maximum number of letters is ten, although it is highly unlikely that even an excellent applicant will have ten strong letters worth sending. Typically, medical schools require a minimum of three letters but request no more than six.

Whom should I ask?

Ideally, at least one letter should be from a professor whose class you were in (typically during college), who can attest to your academic abilities and whether you are likely to be a successful medical student. Furthermore, *it is a large red flag if you did significant scientific research and yet lack a letter from the professor in charge of your laboratory* (also known as the principal investigator or P.I.). Similarly, if you have been involved in some sort of long-term extracurricular activity and highlight it as the cornerstone of your application, then it makes sense to (and may even raise suspicion not to) include a letter from whoever may have supervised or overseen your efforts in that arena. Such an absence may imply to some admissions committee members that you oversold your degree of involvement in the activity, or that your participation ended on a sour note.

In general, your letter writer should be someone who knows you well enough to describe you thoughtfully. If you took a class with 400 students and never spoke to the course instructor or attended office hours, he is unlikely to provide you with much more than a generically nice letter indicating how tough his course was and how your getting an A- was a real accomplishment. However, admissions committees yawn at such banal praise. Your letter-writer should be someone in a good position to speak about at least a few of these considerations:

Important topics in letters of recommendation:

- Unique obstacles you overcame

- Unique attributes you possess that can add to the medical school

- Cognitive abilities, including scientific competency Interpersonal skills, especially communication and leadership

- Ethical values

- Passions, interests, and goals

- Reliability, resilience, capacity for improvement

- Cultural awareness

Another key consideration is how reputable the letter writer is. All things being equal, a letter from a renowned, prize-winning professor carries more clout than, say, a first-year graduate student fresh out of her undergraduate training. An academic physician-scientist whom you did clinical research with during college will impress more than your local private-practice doctor whom you shadowed a couple times over the summer. The well-known head of an international NGO you volunteered with for three straight summers will carry more weight than the pastor of the church youth group you attended during high school.

Many applicants, however, find themselves in a tough situation: of course, they would prefer to get that senior faculty member to write their letter, but they have no real relationship with that individual. Often you can solve the dilemma by having two letter writers collaborate to produce one letter. For instance, if you did research or did the lab portion of a course under the tutelage of a graduate student and never interacted with the P. I. or course professor, then you can ask the graduate student to work with the P.I. or professor to write a comprehensive letter. The graduate student—who best knows you—can inform her about your personal qualities, while the P.I. or professor is ultimately the one who writes and *signs* the letter. In this case, you combine the personal touch of the graduate student with the imprimatur of the senior faculty member. If this hybrid approach is not possible, we generally encourage you to err on the side of getting the letter from the person who knows you best, even if their name or title carries less cachet.

Some applicants find they have a hard time identifying enough letter-writers of any stature who can write an intimate and favorable letter on their behalf. While this may be due to bad circumstances—they may attend a large university where it is truly difficult to get to know one's professors—oftentimes this may be a reflection of the fact that they did not make extra effort to get to know their instructors, or were haphazard in pursuing volunteer work or extracurricular activities. Keep in mind as you enter and go through your undergraduate years that your interpersonal skills and activities play a major role in the quality of your letters of recommendation, and sometimes this requires you to take a more proactive, rather than passive, approach to doing things.

How to ask

To ensure you will receive a strong and timely letter of recommendation, you will need to ask for a letter the right way. After thinking carefully about whom you will ask, you will need to consider how best to make the request. For example, if you are still in college, the best way to ask one of your professors is in person and in private, by appointment, hopefully when they are unhurried and not distracted or in a bad mood. At the face-to-face meeting, you can first bring up that you are applying to medical school with a brief explanation of why you are interested. Indicate that you would be honored if they might consider writing one of your letters of recommendation. Remember to ask whether they think they can write you a *strongly positive* letter (giving them the opportunity to decline if they do not feel this is possible). Ideally, you've asked someone with whom you have a solid rapport, so your request will seem only natural and you will avoid the awkwardness of a polite rejection.

If that person agrees, you should already be prepared to help them produce the best letter possible. To that end, you should come with printed materials that the letter writer can reference. Write down helpful information like your background, activities, and grades, as well as more intangible aspects including your passions, interests, and personal traits. You can discuss why you want to be a doctor, what your professional goals are, and how medical school will best prepare you to achieve your plans for the future (if you have already drafted your personal statement, feel free to include this). Your talking points may turn into the writer's selling points when he or she discusses you in their letter. Your writer may be a busy person who meets dozens of people each day, so they will greatly appreciate whatever materials you provide to help them with these details. In some circumstances, an additional useful touch may be to include a photo of yourself so your writer can remember who you are (and even what gender you are; we've read letters in which a "he" has been called a "she")!

If you know your letter writer very well, you may be able to have a frank discussion about what you would like the letter to say. However, tread with caution, as you may appear overbearing and disrespectful if you seem to demand how your letter should be written.

To have your letters properly submitted to AMCAS, you must also include some other materials. Be sure to include an AMCAS "Letter Request Form" which will have your AMCAS letter ID and AAMC ID printed on it. Both of these IDs must be printed on the letter of recommendation, and the letter must be printed on the official letterhead of the organization to which the letter writer belongs, if any. Let your letter writer know of these requirements early on. You can find the Letter Request Form using your AMCAS application. If it is too early to begin an AMCAS application online, simply wait until later to have your letter writer fill out the form, but have them write the letter anyway and save it. You can have them add the IDs later. Let them know about letter forwarding services, and provide them with information on how to access the service of your choosing. By having all of this information in their hands when you ask them to write a letter, you will appear to be highly organized, professional, and considerate—traits that will make an excellent impression even before your letter writer begins drafting his or her letter.

When to ask

Many applicants make the mistake of asking their letter writers much too late. Other applicants miscalculate how long it will take for their letter writer to follow through and actually complete and submit the letter. Remember: failure to have the letters of recommendation submitted in time may lead to a delay in your application being reviewed, which in turn may lead to compromising your chances of admission. So even though this aspect of the application process may seem out of your control in some ways, do everything you can to stay on top of the situation! Try to find out if your letter writer has a reputation for being slow or tardy. When you ask for a letter of recommendation, be sure to highlight that you need your letter completed by the time you apply. Set a firm date, and politely email them from time to time to remind them of the deadline if you feel your letter writer is procrastinating on your letter. You can explain how important it is for you to apply early, but don't seem too pushy about it.

One reality applicants fail to appreciate is that the best time to ask for a letter is when you know your letter writer the best. Some applicants ask letter writers whom they have only known for a short time. Other students make the mistake of asking for a recommendation from someone they lost contact with many years ago. In these cases, letter writers either have not known you long enough to write a thoughtful letter, or they have forgotten your details and are weaker advocates than they would have been if you had asked them earlier.

The solution to these problems is to ask *for a letter of recommendation at the peak of your relationship with the letter-writer*. This may even be in your freshman or sophomore year, when you have just finished a class in which you have connected with the instructor. This not only increases the likelihood that your letters will not be submitted last-minute, but also ensures your letter-writers are putting pen to paper when you are fresh and favorable in their minds. Create an Interfolio (see above) account that will receive and store your letters of recommendation virtually. This account can hold your letters as you accumulate them throughout your college years. When the time is right, you can then have these letters forwarded to AMCAS or directly to the medical schools.

If it is already late in the application cycle and you have been waitlisted or placed on hold for an interview, you can use new letters of recommendation as a way to update your application and perhaps boost your candidacy. However, the letter should come from someone who represents a new activity that you began pursuing after you submitted your application. Do not send another letter from someone who has already submitted one, unless it contains new information about you. On the whole, *late* letters often do not improve your chances, but they have the possibility of slightly boosting it if the letter is superlative or from a respected figure (e.g., a member of the faculty at the medical school).

Non-traditional students often have a difficult time getting letters of recommendation from the faculty of their undergraduate school. Most schools require a letter from at least one professor, which can be difficult for older students who graduated years ago. In these cases, it may be good to call the medical school admissions office and ask for an exception. You might instead include letters from your bosses at work or leaders of the activities and organizations of which you are a major part.

What is the difference between a good letter and a mediocre one?

Let's face it: almost all the letters of recommendations that admission committee members see are going to be quite strong and consistently filled with praise. The average admissions officer is a veritable expert in superlative phrases, because he has read them all many times over in every possible permutation. It's the Lake Wobegon effect taken to the extreme: at top places, every applicant is not only above average, but is described as amongst the very best students that the college has ever produced.

So how to distinguish one letter from another? Specifically, is there any unique or especially personal aspect about your letter that may help you truly stand out to the admissions officer whose vision is already blurred from reading a hundred of these in one sitting? Conversely, are there letters that vaguely allude to potential concerns, damn with faint praise, or are just so generic as to be virtually worthless or even detrimental to a candidate's chances?

Let's take a look at an example of a mediocre letter of recommendation. While you read it, think about why it is poor:

To the Committee on Admissions,

I am writing to recommend BZ to your medical school. BZ was a student of mine from 2019-2020 for Physics 8A, and, as of the time of writing this letter, is currently my student for Physics 8B. BZ performed well for 8A, earning an A- grade. He is off to a somewhat inauspicious start for the spring semester, with a below-average performance on the first quiz for 8B, but I entirely expect him to rally and do well for the remainder of the course.

BZ makes an effort to attend class regularly and often sits in the front row to ask for clarification when he is confused by a concept during lecture. He is punctual in submitting his assignments and will occasionally even visit me during office hours to discuss his homework and go over questions he missed on his graded assignments. This is especially true on the days leading up to important examinations, when he has come to ask me for additional pre-exam tutoring.

The Physics 8A class ended with a capstone group presentation project that required students to do a literature review on a research topic and present their findings to the class. BZ seemed to be a good team player and his group produced a solid project on the mechanics of roller coasters that nicely met course standards.

As an instructor for introductory physics at my university for 12 years, I have taught a number of pre-medical students who enrolled in the class to meet their requirements for entrance into medical school. BZ fits the mold of most pre-medical students I have instructed: smart, studious, hard-working, and responsible. I believe she has demonstrated all the personality traits, as well sufficient aptitude for the scientific and logical reasoning that is necessary *to be successful in medical school.*

For these reasons, I think BZ would be a solid candidate for entrance into your medical school. Should you have any questions or concerns, please contact me.

Best regards,
Dr. VF

It is clear from this letter that its author has a weak relationship with the student. The professor struggles to write anything personal, unique, or substantial about the applicant. This is not necessarily due to a lack of motivation, but because the professor simply does not know enough about BZ. The applicant made the mistake of asking for a letter from a professor he does not know well, for a class in which he did not particularly set himself apart in any outstanding way.

There are several red flags in this letter, any one of which can hamper this applicant's chances of getting into medical school:

> "He is off to a somewhat inauspicious start for the spring semester, with a below-average performance on the first quiz for 8B..."

Sometimes letter writers, in their attempt to be as honest and thorough as possible, provide a level of detail that includes both positive and negative performances by the student. You can argue whether this is necessary or not; after all, isn't a below-average grade on a small quiz in Physics 8B a relatively minor matter? Absolutely; but the reality is there are so many qualified applicants who have spotless letters, that any negative comment sticks out like a sore thumb. Admissions officers are looking for any excuse to "thin the herd," and may read between the lines and interpret this one sentence as an indication of the applicant's inconsistency.

> **"BZ makes an effort to attend class regularly... He...will occasionally even visit me during office hours to discuss his homework and go over questions he missed on his graded assignments. This is especially true on the days leading up to important examinations..."**

"Makes an effort" to attend class? "Occasionally" visits during office hours? This does not sound like the most diligent of students, even if the professor tries to spin his comments in the most positive light possible. Moreover, BZ sounds like someone who gears up specifically before exams, suggesting he does his work to achieve good grades rather than necessarily being truly engaged in the subject material.

> "He is punctual...a good team player...fits the mold of most pre-medical students...demonstrates sufficient aptitude..."

Talk about damning with faint praise. Compared to applicants who have sterling letters that are effusive with praise, these observations are relatively meager. BZ comes across as fairly ordinary, someone who meets expectations but does not exceed them. Even the laundry list of positive adjectives in the second to last paragraph—smart, studious, hard-working, responsible—could apply to BZ as well as almost every other medical school applicant out there.

> "I believe SHE has demonstrated all the personality traits..."

Believe it or not, we have read letters in which the applicant's gender keeps switching back and forth, or where the entire letter alludes to a female when the applicant is really male (or vice-versa). Whether the letter writer is either too lazy to proof-read or too busy to really keep track, above all, it clearly reflects the fact that he doesn't know the applicant particularly well. On the one hand, this is inexcusable (on the part of the letter-writer), but unfortunately, it ends up reflecting poorly on the applicant himself.

The applicant may have thought the letter was going

to be strong when he asked for it since he got a good grade in Physics 8A and interacted some with the professor during office hours. The fact is, this letter will sink this applicant's chances, right down to the concluding statement that BZ would be a solid candidate for medical school. There are certain code words and phrases that are used in a letter of recommendation; an applicant's being labeled a solid, or good, or above-average candidate may sound reasonable on paper, but this is typically interpreted by admissions committees as, "We can do better"—especially when contrasted with candidates who are described by their professors as "amongst the best I have ever taught," and "in the top 2% of undergraduates I have worked with."

Take a look at an example of an outstanding letter, and see for yourself what makes the difference:

To the Committee on Admissions,

I cannot express enough how enthusiastically I endorse KO for admission to medical school. I first met KO when she was my student in the 2020 fall semester. I was teaching Materials Science 113, which is a pre-requisite course for those majoring in mechanical engineering. The course teaches how various materials deform and handle loads under various kinds of duress.

While most students come to my office hours seeking clarification on homework (or seeking answers to an upcoming exam), KO was different. When she first came to my office hours, she came in to talk about shoes. I was very confused, until she explained she was attempting to design cheap, easy-to-produce, and durable footwear meant for rural, indigent populations in third-world countries. I learned from her how millions of people in the world go barefoot in places where shoes are most necessary. These people suffer from a range of otherwise preventable health conditions, many of which are quite serious. I was impressed by her tenacity, thoughtfulness, creativity, entrepreneurial spirit, and—most of all—her ability to apply what she knows toward a philanthropic cause.

When I thought I could not be more impressed, I was proven wrong when I saw how brilliantly she applied her coursework knowledge to engineer a shoe made of cheap, sustainable, and durable materials and design. When she asked me to help her, I was inspired to do so. In collaboration with her, other faculty, a handful of similarly bright students, and a generous donation from a regional manufacturer, we designed a prototype shoe fit for mass production. In producing this shoe, KO helped found an organization that is currently seeking the wherewithal to mass-produce and distribute these shoes around the world to those who need them most. Working with her in a team, I admired how she used her humility and gracefulness to gain the respect of her peers. She is a natural leader.

Despite being incredibly busy with this endeavor, KO nonetheless found the time to excel in my MS113 class and earned an A-, a difficult grade to achieve in our department. While a handful of students show the extreme intelligence required to earn such a grade, KO is unique in that she shows the ability to apply what she knows toward creative and visionary ends. Her compassion, social awareness, and humanitarian spirit obviously guide her daily life, and she applies her knowledge to achieve her noble goals.

I expect she will continue that way of life as a physician, and it is inevitable she will be the kind of doctor who will change the world on a great scale. KO is a one-of-a-kind, once-in-a-lifetime student. In my 16 years of teaching, she is easily in the top 1 percent of the thousands of students I have taught. Any medical school in the country would be immeasurably fortunate to have her.

Sincerely,
Dr. RQ

OK... KO is clearly a superstar—but the point here is that her accomplishments and abilities are validated by someone externally, someone who knows her well. She has a well-defined and close relationship with her letter-writer, with whom she worked very closely outside of class on a highly impressive and altruistic activity.

This comes across very clearly in her letter:

Unique obstacles you have overcome

> "In producing this shoe, KO helped found an organization that is currently seeking the wherewithal to mass-produce and distribute these shoes around the world to those who need them most."

KO's obstacles are not necessarily difficult socioeconomic or educational circumstances; she herself may come from a privileged background. However, her challenge is one she created for herself on behalf of others: developing a durable, mass-production shoe on a budget. This compelling narrative forms the framework for the bulk of this letter of recommendation.

Unique attributes you possess that add diversity

> "I was impressed by her tenacity, thoughtfulness, creativity, entrepreneurial spirit, and—most of all—her ability to apply what she knows toward a philanthropic cause."

The professor uses specific adjectives to paint a unique picture of KO that distinguishes her nicely from the large pool of other applicants. It is clear to any admissions officer what attributes KO will bring and add to the talent, experience, depth, and breadth of the medical school student body.

Cognitive abilities, including scientific competency

> "Despite being incredibly busy with this endeavor, KO nonetheless found the time to excel in my MS113 class and earned an A-, a difficult grade to achieve in our department. While a handful of students show the extreme intelligence required to earn such a grade, KO is unique in that she shows the ability to apply what she knows toward creative and visionary ends."

KO got the same grade as BZ above, but note how different the A- feels in KO's case in the context of her larger achievements. The professor appropriately does not make KO's grade the centerpiece of his letter, but rather mentions it to highlight how her extracurricular and academic efforts intertwine, rather than cannibalize from one another.

Interpersonal skills, especially communication and leadership

> "Working with her in a team, I admired how she used her humility and gracefulness to gain the respect of her peers and become a natural leader... I know for certain she will continue that way of life as a physician, and it is inevitable she will be the kind of doctor who will change the world on a great scale."

Many schools are looking for students who have more than smarts and an interesting life story—they also want students who can be leaders within the student body and as physicians in patient care, academia, and administration. The letter sets up KO as someone who is likely to be such an individual.

Ethical values, passions, interests, and goals

> "Her compassion, social awareness, and humanitarian spirit obviously guide her daily life, and she applies her knowledge to achieve her noble goals. I know for certain she will continue that way of life as a physician."

The best letters will discuss how the applicant's attributes and goals will set him or her up for success as a medical student and physician. To this end, you should take the opportunity to discuss with your letter writer ahead of time what your plans are for the future, and how medical school will help you achieve those goals.

Top-level superlatives

> "I cannot express enough how enthusiastically I endorse KO... In my 16 years of teaching, she is in the top 1 percent of the thousands of students I have taught... KO is a one-of-a-kind, once-in-a-lifetime student... Any medical school in the country would be immeasurably fortunate to have her as a student."

In the medical school admissions process, outstanding letters are standard—even expected. With what is essentially "praise-inflation," sometimes it becomes difficult to sort out one superlative candidate from another.

Nevertheless, the top-flight descriptors (top 1%, one-of-a-kind, etc.) used in KO's letter seem to ring true especially when following such a detailed, personalized account of her accomplishments. As a general rule of thumb, admissions committee members do take notice of phrases such as "amongst the best," "top 1% (2%/5%)," etc. A candidate described as "outstanding" certainly trumps one who is "highly qualified" or "very good." And a letter writer shouldn't just support your candidacy for medical school; he should do so "enthusiastically" and "without reservation." In the end, though, you can only control so much in what your letter-writer puts in his letter. Focus more on becoming the kind of applicant who *deserves* these kinds of superlatives, and the rest will fall into place.

Summary

- Mediocre and impersonal letters of recommendation can harm your chances of admission, especially at the post-interview stage of admissions.

- Late applications are often due to late letters. Plan early and try to line up your letter-writers ahead of time as much as possible.

- There are two kinds of letters—committee and individual. All letters go through a letter forwarding service before being sent to medical schools.

- Plan on having 3-6 letters, with at least 1-2 from professors who taught you in college. If you have done research, you should try to include a letter from your research supervisor, preferably the principal investigator (P.I.).

- You can choose to waive the confidentiality of a letter and read it before sending it off. However, this can diminish the weight of your letter, so instead we recommend finding other ways to determine which of your letters are strong before you send them.

- When asking someone to write you a letter, always ask if they can write a "strongly positive" letter for you. Come prepared with written materials that can help them write the best and most personalized letter possible. Give them a firm but fair deadline and periodically remind them of that deadline if it becomes imminent.

Chapter VII

When, Where, and How to Apply

For some confused applicants, choosing when and where to apply seems as haphazard as wearing a blindfold and throwing darts at a calendar and map. With such a wide timeframe in which to apply, and with an endless catalog of schools from which to choose, it is not surprising that many applicants lack a strategic game plan in terms of where and when to apply. Little do they realize, by applying early and choosing the right schools, they can dramatically improve their odds of getting into a school—especially ones that fit their particular needs, like cost, location, curriculum, and career interests.

In this chapter, we will cover the ideal schedule for applying during the application cycle, what to do if you fall behind schedule, and what factors to consider when choosing where to apply. For guidance on letters of recommendation, see Chapter 6. Personal statements, school-specific application essays, and the AMCAS activities section are covered in Chapter 5.

HOW TO APPLY

Rather than apply to each school separately, there is a convenient service that allows applicants to fill out a single generic application that is sent out to all the schools to which the applicant applies. This service is run by the American Association of Medical Colleges (AAMC) and is known as the American Medical College Application Service (AMCAS). The AMCAS application is part of the primary application, meaning it is the first application a student sends out to medical schools. After receiving the primary application, medical schools will then ask applicants to fill out a secondary application, which is usually comprised of a series of essay prompts. In this chapter, we will focus our attention on the primary application; refer to Chapter 5 for advice regarding secondary application essays.

The primary application consists of several elements[1]:

The AMCAS application

- The personal statement
  - An essay(up to 5,300-character) that explains why you want to go to medical school
  - MD/PhD applicants have additional essays.

- Your selection of schools to which you will apply

- Your course work and grades

- Send in your official school grade transcripts so the AAMC can verify your self-reported grades and coursework on your AMCAS application. Note that you must tell your undergraduate institution(s) to also send in a completed copy of the AMCAS "Official Transcript Request Form" along with your official transcript.

- Basic biographical data, including parental information, socioeconomic background, race, and schools attended

- Work and activity experiences – A list of your employment and extracurricular activities, including short (1-2 paragraph) descriptions of each activity, with up to 3 selected as "most meaningful" (this designation allows for a slightly longer description)

- Your MCAT score

- Letters of recommendation

> Note: your letters of recommendation and MCAT score are part of your initial submission to medical schools, but you can submit your AMCAS application even if the AAMC has yet to receive your letters or MCAT scores. However, your application to medical school will not be reviewed by medical schools until after they have received all your letters and at least one set of MCAT scores from AMCAS.

A criminal background check

After you have submitted your AMCAS application, the AAMC will personally verify that your self-reported coursework and grades match what your official transcripts say. Only after the application is verified by the AAMC is it sent off to the medical schools of your choosing. This process can take many weeks and significantly delay the submission of your application. This delay is covered later on in this chapter.

WHEN TO APPLY

There are two crucial questions to consider. The first is deciding whether or not your application is strong enough to apply now, or if you need more time to strengthen an underdeveloped application. If you do apply, the second question becomes what month during the application cycle is the best time to submit your application to medical schools.

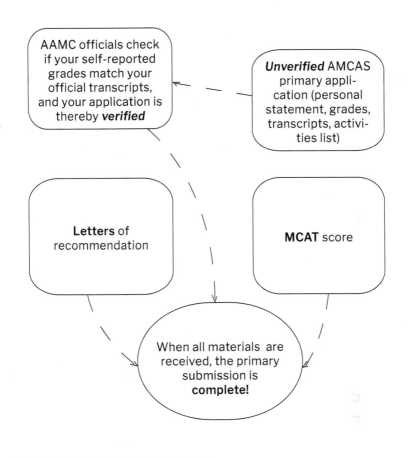

Am I ready to apply—or should I wait?

When you do decide to apply, you should be absolutely sure you are ready. The application process can take hundreds of hours and cost several thousand dollars, so make sure you are a sufficiently competitive applicant that you do not waste precious time and money applying to medical schools to which you have little or no chance of being accepted. Re-applicants are at a disadvantage because they have the additional burden of explaining why they were not accepted to medical school the first time around and why they are now suffi- ciently improved to deserve admission. You want to get in on the first attempt, even if that means (even more) delayed gratification and taking some additional time to bolster your application.

In addition to the primary application requirements listed previously, medical schools require the following from all applicants:

Bachelor's degree (B.A. or B.S.) in any subject from an accredited college or university in the United States or Canada.

Pre-requisite pre-medical courses in college

Some schools will accept Advanced Placement (AP) cred- its in lieu of their corresponding college class. For instance, earning a score of 5 in AP Calculus in college may exempt you from the pre-med requirement of taking a semester of introductory calculus in college. Medical schools vary widely in how they honor AP credit, if at all. Even if AP credit can be used to satisfy some of your pre-requisites, you should not hesitate to enroll in more advanced courses in those sub- jects from which you were exempted, as this may demon- strate your motivation and willingness to accept challenges.

Medical schools vary somewhat in their required courses. Some now require biochemistry or genetics, while others do not. A few—like the University of Southern California, the University of Virginia, and the University of Pennsylvania—have no specific pre-requisite course requirements as of 2020. However, by fulfilling the following list of introductory college courses, you will meet the requirements of the vast majority of medical schools:

- 2 semesters of physics with laboratory sections
- 2 semesters of general biology with laboratory sections
- 2 semesters of general chemistry with laboratory sections
- 2 semesters of organic chemistry with laboratory sections
- 1 semester of calculus
- 2 semesters of writing-intensive courses (English, Comparative Literature, etc.—usually negotiable with broad definition)

An unexpired test score on the Medical College Admissions Test (MCAT). A score is typically valid for 2-3 years, although the precise length depends on the individual school's admissions policy.

While the above items represent the bare minimum requirements necessary to apply to medical school, successful applications contain certain additional features that make them particularly competitive and attractive to admissions committees (read *Chapter 2—"Building your application before and during college"*). Be honest with yourself: if your application has glaring weaknesses or lacks that certain spark, you may not be ready to apply and should strongly consider taking the additional time needed to strengthen your application. For many applicants, this means taking some time off after graduating from college during what are called "gap years." For more information on gap years, read Chapter 4. On the next page is a generalized schedule of a typical traditional applicant who did his pre-med studies during college and applied to medical school in time to start medical school immediately after college. If you are a nontraditional applicant, your schedule will be much different, and it may be helpful to read Chapter 12.

Time	Events
High School *optional*	Shadow physicians, investigate whether pre-medicine and medicine is the right path for you during college. Develop hobbies that demonstrate creativity, leadership, and commitment. Participate in scientific research internships designed by universities for high school students.
College Year 1	Meet with undergraduate premedical advisor and major advisor to devise a multi-year plan to complete your pre-medical and major requirements. Do not overload any one semester, or your grades may suffer. Enroll in or audit classes from different subjects to get an idea of what you want to major in. Explore different clubs and organizations on campus, including community service and health related ones. Some of them should give you direct clinical exposure with patients and physicians.
Summer 1	Summer school to meet requirements, if needed. Summer research/medical programs or intensive volunteering projects (e.g., a summer camp for children with a certain disease or disability).
College Year 2	By the end of this year, complete most of your pre-med classes, especially those tested directly on the MCAT. Begin to consider whom to ask for letters of recommendation and build close personal relationships with those people in anticipation of asking them. Continue your volunteering, research, and club projects, transitioning to taking a creative or leadership position within those projects. Gain more clinical exposure.
Summer 2	Lighten your load to make ample room to focus on studying for the MCAT during your summer. Study intensively for the MCAT with minimized distractions. Take the MCAT right before junior year begins.
College Year 3	Brainstorm and draft your first copy of your personal statement. Find people who can give you feedback for multiple revisions. Ask for letters of recommendation. Get them to be completed by mid-June. Compile a list of schools to apply to. If you haven't taken the MCAT, study and take it before May. Compile a list of schools to apply to. If you haven't taken the MCAT, study and take it before May.

Summer 3	Order official transcripts so they are ready by May 28th. Fill out your AMCAS application and submit it on May 28th. If you are applying to more than 30 schools, pre-write some of your secondary essays by looking up last year's prompts on the Student Doctor Network online forums.
College Year 4	Write and submit your secondary essays no later than two weeks after receiving them. Attend medical school interviews—let your supervisors and teachers know you will be interviewing and need time off (often with little warning) to go interview. Finish degree requirements and continue your volunteering and research projects.
Summer 4	(Hopefully) choose which school to attend by April 30th. Notify the schools you did not choose that you are not attending as soon as your decision has been made (on or before April 30th). Relax (finally).

I'm ready. When is it best to apply during the application season?

Applying to medical schools is like trying to get on all the rides at Disneyland. If you want to beat the lines for the rides, you have to come early at the front gate. If you're late at the front gate, you'll not only take longer to get into the amusement park, but the wait for each ride will be longer as well. By submitting your AMCAS application late, you've let all the other applicants flood across the turnstiles ahead of you. By the time your application has shown up at the schools, many of available interview times may have already been taken, and some of the admission slots even already filled!

The reason submitting early is important is because

most medical schools have a rolling admissions policy. These schools evaluate, interview, and accept applicants on a continuous (rolling) basis throughout the year until the school runs out of available seats. Thus, the later you apply, the fewer open spots there may remain to be filled. One problem is that many applicants have caught on to how important it is to apply early—so now there is even more intense pressure to apply as early as possible, because more and more applicants are doing so.

Box 12: AMCAS Deadlines

As of 2020, these are the main AMCAS application deadlines:

Time	Events
January	2020 Fee Assistance Program (FAP) opens
May 4	AMCAS application opens to be filled out
May 28	**AMCAS application opens for submission**
June 26	AMCAS releases its first batch of verified, submitted applications to medical schools.
August 3	Submission deadline for Early Decision Program (EDP)
September to December	School-specific submission deadlines for primary applications.

The front gate of the admissions process is the AMCAS

Verification process, which begins the moment you hit the "SUBMIT" button that becomes clickable on May 28th for your AMCAS application.

AMCAS Verification

Imagine if you had your entire AMCAS application filled out and ready to go. You hit "submit" thinking you had just sent out your application as early as you thought you could to medical schools.

But then, you learned your application would none-theless be held back for another 40 days so it could be verified by the AAMC. Suddenly, your application is no longer early. This phenomenon happens to thousands of applicants who are unaware of such a delay—which occurs because of the AMCAS transcript verification process.

Figure 1: The Rising Importance of Applying Earlier - AMCAS Verification Times, 2018 - 2019

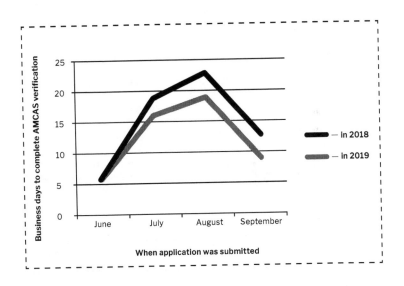

After submitting your AMCAS application, the AAMC verifies that your self-reported grades and coursework match your official transcripts. Because the AAMC only has a limited number of verifiers, this process becomes a clogged bottleneck of too many applicants and not enough reviewers, which can cause untoward delays in some unfortunate cases. Because applications are only sent out after they are verified, there can be a delay of a month, or even longer, before your primary application is actually sent out—which delays everything downstream by at least the same duration.

As shown in the graph above, applicants are heavily

penalized for applying even a month after opening day. In 2019, an applicant who applied on May 29th was verified in fewer than 5 days. On the other hand, an applicant who applied on June 29th took about 28 days to get verified!

Box 13: Early Decision Program (EDP)

The EDP allows applicants to obtain a final admissions decision from participating medical schools by October 1st. By contrast, regular decision programs tend to complete all their final decisions during the spring of the following year.

The advantage of this program is knowing your decision much earlier for, presumably, your dream school. If you are not accepted, you can apply to regular decision programs—but only after October 1st. Furthermore, you can apply to only one school via Early Decision and are required to attend that school if accepted. If you decide to apply via EDP, you must have all primary application materials submitted by August 3rd.

Because participating schools accept so few applicants via EDP, the program is often just as—if not more—selective as regular admissions. Also keep in mind that, if rejected by an EDP, you then have to wait until after October 1st before applying via regular decision, by which time your application will have been submitted relatively late in the game, and will face concomitant disadvantages. Therefore, EDP is a double-edged sword.

Unfortunately for you, many applicants are catching on to the importance of applying early, leading more and more of them to apply earlier each year. This has created an arms race of applying early. The (time) penalty of applying late gets more costly each year, as indicated by the year-by-year trends depicted on the graph.

Because it is so important to submit your AMCAS application on opening day, you should take every step to make sure that you do. Luckily, AMCAS allows you to fill out your AMCAS application a month before opening day, which is the first day you can submit your filled-out application. *Recall that your MCAT scores and letters of recommendation are not required for submission for verification, so do not make the mistake of delaying your submission on account of delayed letters or scores.* You can submit those items later, *after* your AMCAS application has been verified. Many applicants fail to submit their applications for verification in a timely manner. Often this is because they misjudged how long it takes to request and submit official school transcripts to the AAMC. Another reason is that they take too long to draft and revise their personal statements. Plan on requesting your official transcripts immediately after the AMCAS application opens on May 4th, and begin drafting your personal statement months before. If you plan to take the MCAT *after* submitting to AMCAS, you should note that it takes about one month to receive your score after taking your exam. Ideally, you should take your MCAT at the beginning of April. That way, you can know your score by May 4th and make decisions accordingly, well before you are able to submit your application on May 28th.

After submitting your AMCAS application

By submitting your application early, you will be verified earlier, which ensures yours is amongst the first batch of applications sent to medical schools on June 26th. Note that schools will not evaluate you until they also receive your letters of recommendation and MCAT scores. (For tips on how to submit your letters in a timely fashion, see Chapter 6.)

June 26th is also the date when schools will begin evaluating your application to decide whether or not to extend you a secondary application, which tends to include 1-3 essays, each requiring anywhere from a paragraph to 2 pages. You should take no more than 2 weeks to complete these essays. After submitting your secondary application, medical schools will then determine whether to extend you an invitation to interview, which can begin as early as August.

Many schools accept their first interviewees as early as October 15th. Late applicants may only hear their final decisions by as late as March of the following year.

By applying early and interviewing early, you can not only compete for a greater number of available seats, but you also have the potential (and peace of mind) of finding out much earlier in the season that you've been accepted somewhere—if you're lucky!

Box 14: The rules are different for Texas MD schools (TMDSAS)

The medical schools in Texas use a separate admissions system that runs independently of the AAMC and its AMCAS system (except for Baylor University). This system is called TMDSAS. If you want to apply to any of the schools below, you will have to fill out a separate application using TMDSAS. Note that TMDSAS has a similar process to AMCAS, but it runs about one month earlier. That also means Texas public schools begin interviews a bit earlier than the rest of the country.

The TMDSAS system is also unusual in that admissions occur through a matching process similar to that for residencies. A computer algorithm matches your school preference rankings with the schools' preferences rankings for its applicants, to compute a result that optimizes both your preferences and the schools' preferences.[2]

Medical School	Location (TX)	US Rank
UT Galveston	Galveston	X
UT Houston	Houston	X
UT Rio Grande Valley	Edinburg	X
UT San Antonio	San Antonio	55
UT Southwestern	Dallas	26
Texas Tech HSC	Lubbock	90
Texas Tech HSC (Foster)	El Paso	X
Texas A&M	Bryan	74
University of Houston	Houston	X

Don't interview too early

You might assume that an advantage of applying early is that you may be one of the first interviewees at a given medical school—but interviewing extremely early can actually represent a disadvantage! As a general rule of thumb, you do not want to interview within the first two weeks of interviews at a particular school. Admissions committee members are human beings (*really!*) and are just as susceptible to decision-making biases as anyone else. One of those biases is FOMO (fear of missing out), meaning admissions officers may be reluctant to admit too many applicants so early on, thus risking missing out on stronger applicants who apply later in the year.

This does not mean you should not apply early. It just means that if you are offered an extremely early interview date, simply reschedule your interview sometime after the first two weeks that interviews begin at that school. Most schools typically begin interviewing in August and September, although some schools begin interviewing slightly before or after that timeframe. You can find out if you're an early interviewee by checking the school's online application portal, which likely has an online calendar that lists past and future interview dates. If you are still unsure how early you would be as an interviewee, contact the admissions office, or visit the school-specific discussions on the online forums of the Student Doctor Network (http://forums.studentdoctor.net).

Am I applying late? What do I do?

While it is good to submit your AMCAS application in early June and complete your secondary applications in July for the reasons stated above, do not panic if you fall slightly behind that schedule. In fact, you're generally fine if you are interviewing before December—meaning if you submit your AMCAS application in August, you can be verified by September. By the next month, October, you can then ideally receive, complete, and submit your secondary applications. The interview invitations should then start coming in by late October or early November, allowing you to schedule your first set of interviews by or before Thanksgiving.

If you run into obstacles that cause you to apply late, especially if your application is weak or borderline, then your tardiness may potentially—not definitely—hamstring your already marginal chances. If such a situation arises, consider waiting until the following year and use the intervening time to strengthen your application, making sure to apply early the next time around. If you do end up submitting your primary application behind schedule, one helpful trick is to start pre-writing your secondary applications ahead of time while waiting for your AMCAS application to be verified. To find out the types of essay questions beforehand, you can go to the online forums at the Student Doctor Network (http://forums.studentdoctor.net), where the prompts are listed by school. By the time you do receive your secondary applications, you will have already written your essays and can submit your application immediately after receiving it.

You should also take special note of which schools have rolling and non-rolling admissions. At schools with rolling admissions, you will be competing for fewer and fewer available seats as the application season progresses. If you are invited to interview after November, you may even wish to call the admissions office and ask if you are interviewing for a waitlist position only. Realize that they may not give you a straight answer. At non-rolling schools, final admissions decisions are made only after all interviewees have been interviewed. This means, in theory, all applicants have an equal chance of admittance regardless of when their application was processed. If you applied late and have to choose where to interview, it makes sense to prioritize schools with non-rolling admissions. If you don't know whether the school is rolling or not, call or email the admissions office to ask.

WHERE TO APPLY

Many applicants have the credentials to get into medical school, yet lack a sensible strategy in deciding which schools to apply to. As a result, some spend an inordinate amount of time, energy, and money with little to show for at the end; an unfortunate minority wind up not getting accepted anywhere. With these considerations in mind, what general principles should you consider when making this all-important decision?

Err on the side of applying too broadly rather than too narrowly

There are two conflicting realities in applying to medical school:

The first is that you won't have the time or money to apply everywhere. As of 2020, the AAMC charges applicants $170 to send an AMCAS application to his first medical school and $40 per additional school. The vast majority of those schools will ask their applicants to fill out a secondary application, which typically costs an additional $75 to $125. Traveling to interviews tacks on even further major expenses. Moreover, filling out each school's secondary essays can take hours of precious time.

The second reality is that (unless you are a superstar who has her pick of the very best schools), you want to apply to as many medical schools as you can, because the probability of being accepted at any individual medical school is quite low—somewhere around *seven percent*. If you are a solid but not spectacular candidate, especially given the somewhat arbitrary way that medical school admissions decisions are sometimes made, it may be beneficial to apply to a large number of schools to increase your odds of acceptance.

We as admissions faculty try to approach the admissions process with as much fairness and equanimity as possible. However, consider the reality that most medical schools process somewhere between 4,000 to 15,000 applications each year over the course of several months, with the help of dozens of committee members. With so many applicants, admissions faculty, and days in the year, there is tremendous room for variation and inconsistency in how applications are processed. A weak applicant may get in because of luck—perhaps his or her reviewer was in a fantastic and particularly generous mood that day. On the other hand, a strong applicant may not get an interview because his or her hobbies reminded the reviewer of a crazy ex-girlfriend or ex-boyfriend. For most candidates who fall somewhere in the middle of the pack, the *best way to mitigate this kind of variability is to make sure you apply to a sufficiently large number of schools.*

How many schools to apply to?

While it's clear you should apply to more than just a handful of schools, the exact number depends on you. Strong applicants should generally be fine applying to 15-25 schools, while borderline applicants may wish to consider applying to somewhere between 40-60 schools, recognizing that at a certain point costs may become prohibitively expensive. By "borderline," we mean applicants who may barely get into the lowest-ranked MD schools, which typically admit applicants with GPAs in the low- to mid-3 range and MCAT scores ranging from the 63rd to 76th percentiles. Anything below these cut-offs should give you strong reason to consider buffing up your application before applying, because your odds may otherwise be extremely low. (Note that these guidelines may not apply to underrepresented minorities in medicine, who have historically gained admittance with lower MCAT scores and GPAs).

Box 15: Fee Assistance Program (FAP)

As of 2020, the AAMC offers the FAP for applicants whose total income is equal to or less than four times the 2019 poverty level for their family size.

Under FAP, applicants are given valuable services at a reduced or waived price. Participants can take the MCAT at reduced cost and receive free preparation materials valued at about $268.80. Most importantly, applicants can apply to up to 20 medical schools free of charge (a $970 value), with additional schools priced at normal value.[3]

Because the program applies to the MCAT and AMCAS, you should apply for the program before using either service so you can receive benefits for both programs.

If you do apply to a large number of schools, your application process will be expensive and time-consuming. Do the math: applying to 80 schools will cost about $10,000 in anticipated primary and secondary application fees—and that does not even include interview expenses. Most of these schools will require you to write essays about a page-long on average, meaning you may have to write up to 80 high-quality pages of autobiographical prose within the span of 1-2 months—amounting to what may feel like a full-time job. Applying to so many schools should only be a last resort for borderline applicants who may otherwise never get into an MD school in the United States.

You may think applying to 50—or even 30—schools means you are resorting to a shotgun approach and essentially trying to get in anywhere and everywhere. But consider that even if you applied to 65 schools, this still represents fewer than half of the accredited medical schools in the United States. You will need to apply some further criteria to help you strategically eliminate a vast number of medical schools from your list.

Figure out which schools are a good match for you and your credentials

While it's of course good to reach for the stars, a fatal mistake some applicants make is failing to research which schools they are both competitive for and a good match with. You should include on your list a number of schools that have a history of recruiting applicants who match your academic, geographic, socioeconomic, or racial background.

Academic background

Consider first your MCAT and GPA when choosing where to apply. This is why we recommend taking the MCAT in time to receive your scores by May, when you can first begin to assemble your school list in AMCAS. Many (but not all) schools use MCAT scores and GPAs as a first pass to screen applicants, meaning they automatically reject applicants who fail to meet a predetermined (and often undisclosed) threshold.

We recommend splitting your school list into three categories based on whether the school tends to accept students with scores higher, lower, or the same as yours. As a general rule of thumb, *a quarter of your schools should be 'safeties," where the average admitted student has lower scores (although even these cannot be considered guarantees, since other factors invariably come into play). Another quarter should be 'reaches," representing schools comprised of students with generally higher numbers than yours. Finally, the remaining half should be 'matches," in which accepted applicants have scores very similar to yours.*

A tricky part of choosing schools is when your GPA and MCAT scores are quite incongruent—for instance, you own a low GPA and high MCAT score. Sometimes, a high MCAT score can compensate for a low GPA and "average out." A helpful tool to help you average out your GPA and MCAT score is to combine them into one magic number or "**superscore.**"

> *Superscore*=pre 2015 scaled MCAT score+(GPA x 10)

This metric was developed before the introduction of the 2015 MCAT that we have today, so it is based on the old (pre-2015) grading scale and thus requires a reverse score conversion. You can convert your MCAT score to its pre-2015 equivalent by looking at the percentile rank (which should be provided in your score report), and then finding the corresponding pre-2015 MCAT score for that same percentile rank, using the chart provided on the next page.

In general, you can figure out which schools fall into the categories of safeties, reaches, and matches based on the following guidelines:

Safety (25%)	Match (50%)	Reach (25%)
School is -3 or more superscore points from yours	School is ±2 superscore points from yours	School is +3 or more superscore points from yours

For a list of all the US medical (MD) medical schools, including their MCAT, GPA, superscore, and admissions chances, see the comprehensive chart in Figure 2 at the end of this chapter.

A borderline applicant is generally defined as someone whose "match" schools are among the least selective in the nation. Such applicants would not really have any "safety" schools they could feel fairly confident of gaining admission to.

Percentile Rank	Pre-2015 MCAT Score
99.9	45
99.9	44
99.9	43
99.9	42
99.7	41
99.5	40
99.2	39
99	38
98	37
97	36
96	35
94	34
91	33
88	32
83	31
79	30
73	29
67	28
61	27
55	26
49	25
43	24
37	23
32	22
27	21
23	20
19	19
15	18
12	17
10	16
8	15
6	14
5	13
3	12
2	11
2	10
1	9
1	8
0.3	7
0.2	6
0	5
0	4

If you fall into this category, you have three tough choices: (1) go for it, acknowledging that there is a reasonable chance that you may not be accepted anywhere; (2) retake the MCAT, rebuild your GPA, or pursue an intensive extracurricular project, like publishing scientific research or joining the Peace Corps, that will enhance your application a year or two from now; or (3) cast a wider net by applying to Doctor of Osteopathy (DO) or non-U.S. schools, which are somewhat less competitive.

There are disadvantages to each option. For (1), you place yourself at great risk of being rejected everywhere, and as a re-applicant your chances of admissions become worse. For (2), you delay your training and, thereby, your career. With respect to (3), although DO physicians and foreign medical graduates have the same rights and responsibilities as individuals with an MD degree from an American medical school, you should be aware that there is sometimes a stigma associated with these alternative paths that, depending on what your future plans are, may harm your career and employment prospects moving forward. Your unique situation and personality, any time pressures you may feel, how risk-taking or risk-averse you may be, and the degree to which you might care about outward perceptions may each factor into how you decide to proceed.

Geographic location

You can be at a *significant* advantage (or disadvantage)

when applying to public medical schools, because these schools tend to favor in-state residents over applicants who come from a different state. Even some private schools show modest preferences for their in-state residents.

Public schools vary widely in how much they prefer in-state applicants. For instance, in 2020, the University of New Mexico had an acceptance rate of 41.6% for in-state (IS) applicants, but only a 1.6% acceptance rate for out-of-state (OOS) applicants—26 times less! On the other end of the spectrum, the University of Michigan had only a 2x preference for in-state applicants.[4]

As a rule of thumb, you should generally apply to *all your in-state medical schools* no matter what, because you will enjoy a significant boost to your chances by virtue of your home-field advantage. Conversely, you should not spend an inordinate amount of time applying to OOS schools that have a strong preference for in-state residents, unless there is some truly compelling reason why you really want to go there. Note that for states without any public medical schools, there are some neighboring state public schools that often will treat those applicants as in-state residents. An example of this is students from Wyoming, Alaska, Idaho, and Montana, who can apply to the University of Washington as, essentially, in-state applicants.

For more data on this subject, refer to the chart in Figure 3 which shows schools that are somewhat less parochial in regard to accepting OOS applicants.

Alma mater

If your undergraduate institution also has an affiliated medical school, you should apply there. Medical schools often tend to favor applicants who come from their affiliated undergraduate campus.
This is particularly true of Ivy League medical schools— who will also show some favoritism for applicants coming from other Ivy League universities other than their own.

Mutual fit

Some medical schools have specific missions, goals, and emphases. Avoid applying to schools that do not align well with your personal and career interests. The most common special-interest schools are those that are looking for physicians to serve a particular community, and those that have a strong emphasis on research and training physician-scientists.

Box 16: List of new and anticipated medical schools

New medical schools tend to be less selective. These are generally good schools to apply to for applicants with borderline MCAT scores and GPAs. Note that some of these schools may have a preference for in-state residents. California, Texas, and Michigan are the biggest winners in who gains the most medical schools.

Medical School	Starting Year	State
MAYO MEDICAL SCHOOL - ARIZONA	2017	AZ
HACKENSACK MERIDIAN AT SETON HALL	2018	NJ
NYU LONG ISLAND	2019	NY
TCU FORT WORTH SCHOOL OF MED.	2019	TX
UNIVERSITY OF HOUSTON	2020	TX
KAISER PERMANENTE SCHOOL OF MED	2020	CA

The following schools are attempting to begin instruction within the next few years, as of 2014:

Medical School	Starting Year	State
U OF TEXAS - TYLER	?	TX
MARIST HEALTH QUEST SCHOOL OF MED.	2022	NY
ROSEMAN UNIVERSITY	2023	NV

Many schools heavily favor applicants who demonstrate interest and experience in serving underserved communities.

Medical School	NIH funding (2019)
HARVARD UNIVERSITY	$1,652,587,117
UNIVERSITY OF WASHINGTON	$783,477,354
UNIVERSITY OF CALIFORNIA LOS ANGELES	$707,494,950
UNIVERSITY OF PENNSYLVANIA	$700,452,348
JOHNS HOPKINS UNIVERSITY	$663,031,818
UNIVERSITY OF CALIFORNIA SAN FRANCISCO	$611,867,916
COLUMBIA UNIVERSITY	$585,732,348
CORNELL UNIVERSITY	$582,051,164
WASHINGTON UNIVERSITY IN ST. LOUIS	$564,472,381
DUKE UNIVERSITY	$547,220,193
NEW YORK UNIVERSITY	$542,415,562
UNIVERSITY OF PITTSBURGH	$541,509,000
MAYO CLINIC SCHOOL OF MEDICINE	$512,096,226
UNIVERSITY OF MICHIGAN – ANN ARBOR	$499,633,831
ICAHN SCHOOL OF MED. AT MT. SINAI	$476,578,412
STANFORD UNIVERSITY	$462,489,179
YALE UNIVERSITY	$435,613,678
NORTHWESTERN UNIVERSITY	$434,648,017
VANDERBILT UNIVERSITY	$412,277,266
UNIVERSITY OF CALIFORNIA SAN DIEGO	$408,357,131
BAYLOR COLLEGE OF MEDICINE	$346,416,640

UNIVERSITY OF CHICAGO	$327,066,880
CASE WESTERN RESERVE UNIVERSITY	$323,489,842
EMORY UNIVERSITY	$301,269,278
UNIVERSITVE OF NORTH CAROLINA – CHAPEL HILL	$300,494,476
OREGON HEALTH AND SCIENCE UNIVERSITY	$293,149,537
BOSTON UNIVERSITY	$291,867,425
UNIVERSIY OF WISCONSIN – MADISON	$275,000,000

Certain programs within larger medical schools have their own admissions process and preferences. For instance, the Charles Drew/UCLA program, part of UCLA Medical School, only accepts applicants with a record of helping the underserved. The historically black colleges and universities (HBCUs) also have the similar emphasis and admissions criteria for their own schools. Other schools are research powerhouses and prioritize applicants with strong research experience. Even applicants with stellar grades and MCAT scores will sometimes not gain admittance to these schools, unless they also have laboratory experience, posters, and/or publications. One way to estimate which schools are research-heavy is to look at the schools that receive the most research money from the National Institute of Health. A historical list of the top-ranked medical schools is provided in Figure 4.

Schools you want to go to: Following your heart

After taking all pragmatic and rational factors into consideration, there is simply the matter of following your heart that we do not want you to discount. For instance, you might fantasize about attending Columbia because you like the idea of jogging through Central Park in the morning before lecture starts. Or you fancy the idea of going to UC San Francisco to see the Golden Gate Bridge cresting above a dome of clouds while you study in the campus library. While it is fun—and advisable—to apply to a few dream schools, just make sure to keep your head below the clouds, and not limit yourself or overly idealize any one school that you will be devastated if you do not get into.

Don't forget these other important considerations!

The following aspects of medical school may or may not necessarily be foremost on your radar screen when deciding where to apply. Whatever the case, don't discount their significance—each of these factors can very much affect your enjoyment and experience of the next four years of your life.

- Grading system

    Inquire if the school has grades during its preclinical years. During the first 1-2 years of medical school, students take basic and clinical science courses. These classes may have grades (High Honors/Honors/Pass/Fail, for instance), or there may simply be a Pass/Fail designation. The latter obviously makes medical school significantly less stressful because it obviates competition between students and tampers down the "gunner" mentality that can sometimes be prevalent in highly competitive environments. Beware that some medical schools have a ranked Pass/Fail system, meaning your test scores are collected by the administration to rank you against your peers in later evaluations. Some schools do award honors for exceptional performance during clinical rotations.

- Problem-Based Learning (PBL) and Team-Based Learning

    Many schools are increasing the amount of problem-based learning students do during their preclinical years. This form of learning is quickly replacing lectures as a way to learn class material. In PBL, students are given a fictional case of a patient with symptoms. Students work together to diagnose the patient and devise a treatment plan. Often the students will need to do their own independent research and learn to achieve these goals.

- Students who enjoy active and group learning may prefer schools with PBL-heavy curricula,

214 _ _ _ Insider's Pre-Med Guidebook

while those who prefer and learn better from formal didactic lectures may wish to seek schools which still rely on this more traditional format.

Keep in mind that many schools are in the process of switching over to PBL formats, so be sure to inquire at each school to which you apply about their present and future curricula.

- Length of curriculum
  - Many schools are transitioning to a condensed preclinical curriculum. Traditionally, medical students learned their basic and clinical sciences for two years before going to the hospital to do their clinical rotations. Now, some schools are condensing the preclinical curriculum to 18—or even 12—months, with a greater clinical emphasis right from day 1 of medical school.

- Hospitals, patients, and clinical exposure
  - Clinical exposure during medical school, aside from formal clinical rotations, can consist of volunteer-driven free clinics, structured mentorships with clinicians, and classes meant to build clinical skills by interacting with real patients before you begin your clinical rotations in teaching hospitals.
  - Some students prefer to work with certain socioeconomic, racial, cultural, or geographic communities—which may be well or poorly represented at the university-affiliated hospitals.

Location

Having emotional support may be important during the stressful times you will endure as a medical student. This may mean choosing a school that is closer to your family or friends. There may be practical or financial reasons why this is necessary as well.

Cost

Examine the school's average indebtedness, which can be a more accurate reflection of the school's real cost. Many top-tier private schools have a pricey tuition, but their generous endowment allows them to give generous merit- and need-based financial aid to even upper-middle class students. State schools typically offer subsidized tuition for state residents.

If your family makes over $200,000 a year, has substantial assets (properties, investments, retirement accounts, savings), and if you have few or no siblings in college, you are less likely to receive need-based aid, which would make attending a private school more expensive to attend. A typical private school has a cost of attendance (i.e., living expenses and tuition) at around $85,000 per year, while a public one may be closer to $60,000 per year if you are an in-state resident.

Your future

Many schools have a reputation for sending its graduates to particularly prestigious residency programs and fellowships or to ones in a certain geographic area.

Choose a school that has a history of sending graduates to the programs you may want to be in later in your career. You can get an idea of a school's residency placements by viewing their match list, which is a record of where its graduates have gone onto residency.

Box 17: Applying to the wrong places, a surfer's wipe-out application cycle

J.T. grew up in Cardiff-by-the-Sea, CA, a small surfing community in San Diego County. He loved to rock climb and—most of all—surf. J.T. figured he would want to continue his water-riding hobby as a medical student, so he only applied to medical schools that were close to the gnarliest coastal waves.

J.T. only applied to ten schools, including UCLA, UC San Diego, UC Irvine, USC, University of Miami, and other Florida schools. He was bummed when he did not get accepted to any of those schools. Not only did he apply to too few schools, but also, he ignored the high MCAT, high GPA, and in-state preferences that many of these schools had.

J.T. did some volunteering and research, then reapplied the next year to a more strategic and broad set of schools. He ended up attending Rush Medical College in Chicago, where the waves on Lake Michigan are totally bogus.

Summary

- The primary application consists of your MCAT score(s), letters of recommendation, official college transcripts, and your AMCAS application—which includes your personal statement essay, a list of your extracurricular activities, demographic data, the list of schools your applying to, and your self-reported courses and grades.

- The primary application can be filled out beginning on May 4th and can be sent out beginning May 28th.

AMCAS applications are verified by the AAMC before they are sent to medical schools. This verification process can lead to significant delay in your application being sent out (sometimes by over a month) due to backlogging. Therefore, you should plan to submit your application in the beginning of June rather than waiting too long beyond that. Remember that you can submit your AMCAS application without your MCAT scores and letters of recommendation (but you will need to send them in eventually).

If possible, try to avoid interviewing during the first two weeks of a school's interview season. That exception aside, the earlier you interview, the better your chances, so try to get most of your interviews completed by December.

Especially if you are a borderline applicant, applying late may hurt your odds and increase the likelihood that you will be rejected everywhere. You should try to avoid being a re-applicant, which carries with it some stigma.

If you are a borderline applicant, apply broadly to somewhere between 40-60 schools. If you are a strong applicant, 15-25 should be fine. Remember, there is an element of chance and some arbitrariness in the whole medical school admissions process.

Apply to a good mix of safety, match, and reach schools, based on your GPA and MCAT scores combined. Compare your scores to those of the average admitted applicant at each school. A list of schools is provided in the following figures.

- Recognize the advantages you have as an in-state resident by making sure to apply to your state school(s). Only apply to out-of-state public schools that are amenable to out-of-state residents (see the appendices for a list of such schools).

- To eliminate schools from your list, consider carefully what features and standards you want in a school. Curriculum, cost, location, and your ultimate career goals are each important considerations.

---

[1] https://students-residents.aamc.org/applying-medical-school/faq/what-parts-your-application-tell-medical-schools-2/

[2] http://tmdsas.com/about/TMDSAS_schools.html

[3] https://students-residents.aamc.org/applying-medical-school/article/what-are-benefits-fee-assistance-program/

[4] https://www.accepted.com/medical/in-state-out-of-state-admis

Figure 1:
https://students-residents.aamc.org/content/downloadable/2270/

Figures 2 &3:
https://www.aamc.org/system/files/2019-11/2019_FACTS_Table_A-1.pdf
https://www.shemmassianconsulting.com/blog/average-gpa-and-mcat-score-for-every-medical-school
https://aamc-orange.global.ssl.fastly.net/production/media/filer_public/d9/04/d904b7f4-c3d0-4469-aed1-e5afff500d05/mcat_total_and_section_score_percentile_ranks_2020_for_web.pdf
https://www.usnews.com/best-graduate-schools/top-medical-schools/research-rankings

Figure 4:
  https://www.usnews.com/best-graduate-schools/top-medical-
  schools/research-rankings

NIH funding:
  https://www.usnews.com/best-graduate-schools/top-medical-
  schools/most-research-money-rankings

Figure 2: Compiled list of medical (MD) schools in the United States, 2020

In-State Preference Terms:	Meaning:
Very High	There are 5x or more out of state (OOS) matriculants than in-state (IS) matriculants
High	There are 3-5x OOS matriculants than IS matriculants
Average	1-3x (~2 is the average)
Low	.25-1x
Very Low	<.25x

Figure 2: Compiled list of medical (MD) schools in the United States, 2014

School Name	State	GPA	MCAT Percentile	Super Score	Rep. Rank (USNWR)	# of Applicants	% of IS App.	% of OOS App.	# of Matriculants	% of IS Matric.	% of OOS Matric.	OOS/IS Matric. Likelihood Rating
Albany Medical College	NY	3.6	80	67	X	10,247	18.2%	81.8%	139	28.1%	71.9%	Average
Baylor	TX	3.93	96	75	22	6,688	27.5%	72.5%	186	79.6%	20.4%	Low
Boston University	MA	3.69	94	72	29	9,151	9.2%	90.8%	160	23.8%	76.3%	High
Brown	RI	3.82	91	72	38	7.770	1.2%	98.8%	144	11.1%	88.9%	Very High
California North-state	CA	3.6	82	68	X	4,184	62.2%	37.8%	96	90.6%	9.4%	Very Low
California University	CA	3.66	87	70	X	5,494	50.3%	49.7%	98	83.7%	16.3%	Very Low
Case Western Reserve	OH	3.78	96	74	24	7,556	10.9%	89.1%	214	19.6%	80.4%	High
Central Michigan	MI	3.7	77	68	X	7,360	18.4%	81.6%	103	82.5%	17.5%	Very Low
City College of New York (CUNY)	NY	X	X	X	X	75	100.0%	0.0%	75	100.0%	0.0%	Very Low
Columbia	NY	3.91	98	77	6	7,855	16.3%	83.7%	138	16.7%	83.3%	High

College	State	GPA										Rating
Commonwealth Med. College	PA	3.63	80	67	X	5,781	16.1%	83.9%	115	71.3%	28.7%	Low
Cooper Rowan	NJ	3.75	82	70	94-122	6,826	18.3%	81.7%	111	74.8%	25.2%	Low
Cornell	NY	3.88	96	75	11	6,385	19.5%	80.5%	106	26.4%	73.6%	Average
Creighton	NE	3.77	82	70	X	6,375	2.5%	97.5%	166	6.6%	93.4%	Very High
Darmouth	NH	3.66	89	70	50	8,399	1.1%	98.9%	92	5.4%	94.6%	Very High
Drexel	PA	3.64	85	68	84	14,067	8.3%	91.7%	254	30.7%	69.3%	Average
Duke	NC	3.88	97	76	12	6,951	7.8%	92.2%	121	17.4%	82.6%	High
East Carolina University (Brody)	NC	3.65	74	67	94-122	1,075	99.3%	0.7%	86	100.0%	0.0%	Very Low
East Tennessee State	TN	3.7	67	66	94-122	2,386	26.8%	73.2%	72	90.3%	9.7%	Very Low
Eastern Virginia	VA	3.56	82	68	94-122	6,389	16.8%	83.2%	151	51.7%	48.3%	Low
Einstein	NY	3.81	91	72	40	8,088	20.3%	79.7%	183	47.0%	53.0%	Average
Emory	GA	3.7	89	70	24	10,382	7.7%	92.3%	138	29.7%	70.3%	Average
Florida Atlantic	FL	3.68	85	69	94-122	3,586	60.8%	39.2%	66	42.4%	57.6%	Average

School Name	State	GPA	MCAT Percentile	Super Score	Rep. Rank (USNWR)	# of Applicants	% of IS App.	% of OOS App.	# of Matriculants	% of IS Matric.	% of OOS Matric.	OOS/IS Matric. Likelihood Rating
Florida International University	FL	3.71	74	67	94-122	4,672	53.4%	46.6%	122	81.1%	18.9%	Very Low
Florida State University	FL	3.7	67	66	94-122	7,313	38.0%	62.0%	120	96.7%	3.3%	Very Low
George Washington University	DC	3.7	87	70	58	14,997	0.5%	99.5%	184	3.3%	96.7%	Very High
Georgetown	DC	3.63	85	68	44	13,149	0.5%	99.5%	203	3.4%	96.6%	Very High
Hackensack Meridian	NJ	3.77	82	70	X	4,654	24.6%	75.4%	91	63.7%	36.3%	Low
Harvard	MA	3.9	97	76	1	7,613	7.6%	92.4%	165	11.5%	88.5%	Very High
Hofstra	NY	3.78	93	72	70	5,316	30.3%	69.7%	99	54.5%	45.5%	Low
Howard (HBC)	DC	3.42	53	61	94-122	9,093	0.5%	99.5%	119	5.0%	95.0%	Very High
Indiana University	IN	3.75	80	69	47	6,683	10.6%	89.4%	365	78.1%	21.9%	Low
Jefferson	PA	3.71	89	70	57	9,443	11.3%	88.7%	270	32.2%	67.8%	Average
Johns Hopkins	MD	3.81	99	76	2	6,016	6.1%	93.9%	120	12.5%	87.5%	Very High

Kaiser Permanente	CA	X	X	X	X	X	X	X	X	X	X
Loma Linda	CA	3.82	80	69	X	6,318	37.2%	62.8%	168	43.5%	56.5%	Average
Louisiana State (New Orleans)	LA	3.68	77	68	X	3,827	18.9%	81.1%	198	91.9%	8.1%	Very Low
Louisiana State (Shreveport)	LA	3.65	64	66	94-122	2,866	23.9%	76.1%	150	90.0%	10.0%	Very Low
Loyola Chicago	IL	3.5	74	65	88	14,905	11.4%	88.6%	170	34.1%	65.9%	Average
Marshall	WV	3.6	57	63	X	2,205	8.4%	91.6%	80	78.8%	21.3%	Low
Mayo	MN	3.92	98	76	6	7,265	6.3%	93.7%	102	5.9%	94.1%	Very High
Medical College of Georgia	GA	3.8	82	70	84	3,100	40.4%	59.6%	230	97.0%	3.0%	Very Low
Medical College of Wisconsin	WI	3.78	80	69	X	7,936	9.3%	90.7%	252	54.8%	45.2%	Low
Medical University of S. Carolina	SC	3.7	80	68	58	4,088	15.2%	84.8%	171	87.7%	12.3%	Very Low

School Name	State	GPA	MCAT Percentile	Super Score	Rep. Rank (USNWR)	# of Applicants	% of IS App.	% of OOS App.	# of Matriculants	% of IS Matric.	% of OOS Matric.	OOS/IS Matric. Likelihood Rating
Meharry (HBC)	TN	3.5	53	62	X	7,381	4.1%	95.9%	114	19.3%	80.7%	High
Mercer	GA	3.72	70	67	X	1,122	100.0%	0.0%	120	100.0%	0.0%	Very Low
Michigan State (MD Program)	MI	3.71	74	67	X	7,994	20.3%	79.7%	190	74.2%	25.8%	Low
Missouri - Kansas City	MO	3.7	64	66	88	1,303	20.1%	79.9%	115	64.3%	35.7%	Low
Morehouse (HBC)	GA	3.65	67	66	X	7,316	11.2%	88.8%	100	55.0%	45.0%	Low
Mount Sinai	NY	3.87	97	76	20	6,592	21.2%	78.8%	140	31.4%	68.6%	Average
New York Medical College	NY	3.6	87	69	94-122	12,714	17.1%	82.9%	215	51.2%	48.8%	Low
New York University (NYU)	NY	3.93	99	77	4	8,937	15.9%	84.1%	103	21.4%	78.6%	High
Northeast Ohio Med. University	OH	3.71	77	68	X	4,069	26.1%	73.9%	151	83.4%	16.6%	Very Low
Northwestern University	IL	3.91	98	76	18	6,878	12.3%	87.7%	159	32.1%	67.9%	Average

University	State	GPA										
Nova Southeastern University	FL	3.64	82	68	X	5,120	37.4%	62.6%	51	58.8%	41.2%	Low
NYU Long Island	NY	X	X	X	X	2,390	24.5%	75.5%	24	58.3%	41.7%	Low
Oakland	MI	3.8	77	69	X	7,550	19.5%	80.5%	125	53.6%	46.4%	Low
Ohio State	OH	3.79	89	71	34	7,725	16.8%	83.2%	209	53.6%	46.4%	Low
Oregon Health and Science	OR	3.65	77	68	28	6,209	8.7%	91.3%	160	73.1%	26.9%	Low
Pennsylvania State-Hershey	PA	3.77	82	70	X	11,827	9.9%	90.1%	152	36.8%	63.2%	Average
Ponce Health Sciences University	PR	3.65	43	62	X	1,525	35.0%	65.0%	100	79.0%	21.0%	Low
Quinnipiac	CT	3.6	85	68	94-122	7,701	5.4%	94.6%	94	25.5%	74.5%	Average
Rosalind Franklin	IL	3.45	64	64	X	15,415	10.1%	89.9%	189	52.4%	47.6%	Low
Rush	IL	3.58	85	68	58	11,297	13.3%	86.7%	144	22.9%	77.1%	High
Rutgers (Biomed. & Health Sci.)	NJ	3.68	89	70	70	5,112	29.5%	70.5%	178	80.9%	19.1%	Very Low

School Name	State	GPA	MCAT Percentile	Super Score	Rep. Rank (USNWR)	# of Applicants	% of IS App.	% of OOS App.	# of Matriculants	% of IS Matric.	% of OOS Matric.	OOS/IS Matric. Likelihood Rating
Rutgers (Robert Wood Johnson)	NJ	3.64	85	68	74	5,689	26.4%	73.6%	165	76.4%	23.6%	Low
Southern Illinois	IL	3.7	67	66	X	1,196	94.6%	5.4%	72	100.0%	0.0%	Very Low
St. Louis University	MO	3.84	87	71	74	6,834	6.7%	93.3%	180	18.9%	81.1%	High
Stanford	CA	3.89	97	76	4	7,506	32.6%	67.4%	90	37.8%	62.2%	Average
Stony Brook University (SUNY)	NY	3.8	91	72	58	5,241	41.4%	58.6%	136	79.4%	20.6%	Low
SUNY Downstate	NY	3.75	89	71	X	5,761	42.0%	58.0%	200	89.5%	10.5%	Very Low
SUNY Syracuse		3.67	85	69	84	4,482	47.5%	52.5%	169	79.3%	20.7%	Low
TCU and UNTHSC	TX	3.62	74	66	X	1,393	54.6%	45.4%	60	51.7%	48.3%	Low
Temple University	PA	3.75	85	70	66	11,509	10.3%	89.7%	195	46.2%	53.8%	Average
Texas A&M	TX	3.84	85	70	74	5,151	78.9%	21.1%	120	94.2%	5.8%	Very Low

School	State	GPA										
Texas Tech Health Sci. (El Paso)	TX	3.7	74	66	X	4,882	80.7%	19.3%	180	89.4%	10.6%	Very Low
Texas Tech Health Sci. (Lubbock)	TX	3.87	85	71	90	4,424	82.5%	17.5%	104	89.4%	10.6%	Very Low
Tufts	MA	3.66	89	70	53	12,764	7.9%	92.1%	200	21.0%	79.0%	High
Tulane	LA	3.52	77	66	X	12,982	3.5%	96.5%	190	19.5%	80.5%	High
UC Davis	CA	3.7	82	69	40	7,161	65.1%	34.9%	123	99.2%	0.8%	Very Low
UC Irvine	CA	3.78	91	72	44	6,281	71.5%	28.5%	104	85.6%	14.4%	Very Low
UC Riverside	CA	3.72	80	68	91	5,902	71.5%	28.5%	77	100.0%	0.0%	Very Low
UC San Diego	CA	3.77	93	72	21	7,398	57.0%	43.0%	134	85.8%	14.2%	Very Low
UC San Francisco	CA	3.8	94	73	6	7,900	44.8%	55.2%	171	77.8%	22.2%	Low
UCLA	CA	3.85	94	74	6	13,101	44.0%	56.0%	180	62.2%	37.8%	Low
UNC Chapel Hill	NC	3.66	85	69	23	7,383	15.0%	85.0%	190	87.4%	12.6%	Very Low
Uniformed Services (Hebert)	MD	3.64	74	66	X	3,096	6.2%	93.8%	175	8.6%	91.4%	Very High

School Name	State	GPA	MCAT Percentile	Super Score	Rep. Rank (USNWR)	# of Applicants	% of IS App.	% of OOS App.	# of Matriculants	% of IS Matric.	% of OOS Matric.	OOS/IS Matric. Likelihood Rating
Universidad Central del Caribe	PR	3.77	43	63	X	1,170	43.4%	56.6%	75	89.3%	10.7%	Very Low
University at Buffalo (SUNY)	NY	3.64	80	67	79	3,823	51.1%	48.9%	180	82.8%	17.2%	Very Low
University of Alabama	AL	3.77	77	69	31	4,373	11.5%	88.5%	186	85.5%	14.5%	Very Low
University of Arizona	AZ	3.72	77	68	65	9,940	8.0%	92.0%	119	79.0%	21.0%	Low
University of Arizona (Phoenix)	AZ	3.77	85	70	X	5,835	13.4%	86.6%	80	61.3%	38.8%	Low
University of Arkansas	AR	3.78	70	68	81	2,566	14.0%	86.0%	172	91.3%	8.7%	Very Low
University of Central Florida	FL	3.79	87	71	84	5,120	47.1%	52.9%	120	67.5%	32.5%	Low
University of Chicago	IL	3.84	97	75	17	5,683	11.9%	88.1%	90	21.1%	78.9%	High

University		GPA										Rating
University of Cincinnati	OH	3.75	91	72	44	4,734	25.9%	74.1%	185	52.4%	47.6%	Low
University of Colorado	CO	3.76	83	70	31	8,666	8.8%	91.2%	182	47.3%	52.7%	Average
University of Connecticut	CT	3.77	77	69	53	3,286	16.4%	83.6%	110	76.4%	23.6%	Low
University of Florida	FL	3.79	89	71	40	4,499	52.2%	47.8%	137	87.6%	12.4%	Very Low
University of Hawaii	HI	3.76	82	70	62	1,980	12.6%	87.4%	77	84.4%	15.6%	Very Low
University of Houston	TX	3.81	87	71		X	X	X	X	X	X	X
University of Illinois	IL	3.6	85	68	55	5,722	31.9%	68.1%	291	79.4%	20.6%	Low
University of Iowa	IA	3.81	89	71	34	3,878	8.9%	911%	152	64.5%	35.5%	Low
University of Kansas	KS	3.85	80	70	62	3,207	15.6%	84.4%	211	86.7%	13.3%	Very Low

School Name	State	GPA	MCAT Percentile	Super Score	Rep. Rank (USNWR)	# of Applicants	% of IS App.	% of OOS App.	# of Matriculants	% of IS Matric.	% of OOS Matric.	OOS/IS Matric. Likelihood Rating
University of Kentucky	KY	3.84	70	68	68	2,394	23.4%	76.6%	203	89.2%	10.8%	Very Low
University of Louisville	KY	3.68	74	67	78	3,848	14.0%	86.0%	162	73.5%	26.5%	Low
University of Maryland	MD	3.8	85	70	34	5,185	17.8%	82.2%	148	62.2%	37.8%	Low
University of Massachusetts	MA	3.77	89	71	47	4,094	25.5%	74.5%	162	69.8%	30.2%	Low
University of Miami	FL	3.72	87	70	50	9,175	23.9%	76.1%	207	56.5%	43.5%	Low
University of Michigan	MI	3.78	89	71	15	7,896	15.7%	84.3%	177	41.2%	58.8%	Average
University of Minnesota	MN	3.71	85	69	40	5,561	16.7%	83.3%	240	85.4%	14.6%	Very Low
University of Mississippi	MS	3.7	60	65	X	428	99.8%	0.2%	165	100.0%	0.0%	Very Low

University	State	GPA										
University of Missouri	MO	3.75	77	69	79	3,390	17.6%	82.4%	240	85.4%	14.6%	Very Low
University of Nebraska	NE	3.75	91	72	62	1,590	18.6%	81.4%	132	86.4%	13.6%	Very Low
University of Nevada (Las Vegas)	NV	3.6	74	66	X	1,942	14.4%	85.6%	60	88.3%	11.7%	Very Low
University of Nevada (Reno)	NV	3.74	77	68	94-122	1,484	18.9%	81.1%	68	89.7%	10.3%	Very Low
University of New Mexico	NM	3.74	67	66	81	1,862	13.1%	86.9%	103	98.1%	1.9%	Very Low
University of North Dakota	ND	3.5	70	65	X	1,718	8.8%	91.2%	77	61.0%	39.0%	Low
University of Oklahoma	OK	3.7	77	68	70	2,662	15.8%	84.2%	165	93.3%	6.7%	Very Low
University of Pennsylvania	PA	3.89	98	76	3	6,578	9.2%	90.8%	150	20.7%	79.3%	High
University of Pittsburgh	PA	3.75	94	73	14	7,013	11.8%	88.2%	147	35.4%	64.6%	Average

School Name	State	GPA	MCAT Percentile	Super Score	Rep. Rank (USNWR)	# of Applicants	% of IS App.	% of OOS App.	# of Matriculants	% of IS Matric.	% of OOS Matric.	OOS/IS Matric. Likelihood Rating
University of Puerto Rico	PR	3.77	57	65	X	771	52.7%	47.3%	109	94.5%	5.5%	Very Low
University of Rochester	NY	3.7	89	70	34	5,803	22.4%	77.6%	102	27.5%	72.5%	Average
University of South Alabama	AL	3.6	70	66	X	1,554	27.7%	72.3%	74	87.8%	12.2%	Very Low
University of South Carolina	SC	3.6	67	65	91	3,006	17.2%	82.8%	97	76.3%	23.7%	Low
University of South Carolina (Greenville)	SC	3.7	77	68	X	3,582	15.5%	84.5%	105	66.7%	33.3%	Low
University of South Dakota	SD	3.81	77	69	X	836	18.4%	81.6%	70	82.9%	17.1%	Very Low
University of South Florida	FL	3.76	91	72	47	5,574	43.7%	56.3%	182	64.3%	35.7%	Low
University of Southern California	CA	3.7	94	72	31	8,041	47.9%	52.1%	186	82.3%	17.7%	Very Low

University of Tennessee	TN	3.7	80	68	74	2,207	33.3%	66.7%	170	89.4%	10.6%	Very Low
University of Toledo	OH	3.67	77	68	94-122	5,411	23.6%	76.4%	175	76.0%	24.0%	Low
University of Utah	UT	3.84	89	71	38	3,850	14.9%	85.1%	125	79.2%	20.8%	Low
University of Vermont	VT	3.73	80	68	66	6,759	1.5%	98.5%	122	27.0%	73.0%	Average
University of Virginia	VA	3.84	96	74	29	4,790	17.1%	82.9%	156	43.6%	56.4%	Average
University of Washington	WA	3.75	80	69	13	8,190	12.6%	87.4%	270	51.9%	48.1%	Low
UT Austin	TX	3.74	87	70	X	5,078	77.9%	22.1%	50	94.0%	6.0%	Very Low
UT Galveston	TX	3.93	85	71	X	5,220	79.3%	20.7%	230	97.0%	3.0%	Very Low
UT San Antonio	TX	3.82	93	72	55	5,299	78.0%	22.0%	211	86.3%	13.7%	Very Low
UT Southwestern	TX	3.84	91	72	26	5,401	75.0%	25.0%	220	86.4%	13.6%	Very Low
UW Madison	WI	3.77	87	71	27	4,815	14.2%	85.8%	179	66.5%	33.5%	Low

School Name	State	GPA	MCAT Percentile	Super Score	Rep. Rank (USNWR)	# of Applicants	% of IS App.	% of OOS App.	# of Matriculants	% of IS Matric.	% of OOS Matric.	OOS/IS Matric. Likelihood Rating
Vanderbilt	TN	3.9	98	76	18	5,982	5.1%	94.9%	97	13.4%	86.6%	Very Low
Virginia Common-wealth	VA	3.7	85	69	68	7,998	14.0%	86.0%	184	56.0%	44.0%	Low
Virginia Tech Carilion	VA	3.51	85	67	81	4,483	16.6%	83.4%	43	20.9%	79.1%	High
Wake Forest	NC	3.67	87	70	52	10,703	8.7%	91.3%	145	31.0%	69.0%	Average
Washington University (STL)	MO	3.89	98	76	58	4,766	4.3%	95.7%	101	11.9%	88.1%	Very High
Wayne State University	MI	3.7	80	68	70	9,993	17.2%	82.8%	292	61.6%	38.4%	Low
West Virginia University	WV	3.8	77	69	84	5,559	3.8%	96.2%	112	59.8%	40.2%	Low
Western Michigan	MO	3.69	X	X	X	4,143	27.5%	72.5%	84	34.5%	65.5%	Average
Wright State	OH	3.61	70	66	94-122	6,119	20.7%	79.3%	119	60.5%	39.5%	Low
Yale	CT	3.9	98	77	15	5,776	4.3%	95.7%	104	15.4%	84.6%	Very High

Figure 3: Schools that are favorable for out-of-state applicants

In-State Preference Terms:	Meaning:
Very High	There are 5x or more out of state (OOS) matriculants than in-state (IS) matriculants
High	There are 3-5x OOS matriculants than IS matriculants
Average	1-3x (~2 is the average)
Low	.25-1x
Very Low	<.25x

Figure 3: Schools that are favorable for out-of-state applicants

School Name	State	GPA	MCAT Percentile	Super Score	Rep. Rank (USNWR)	# of Applicants	% of IS App.	% of OOS App.	# of Matriculants	% of IS Matric.	% of OOS Matric.	OOS/IS Matric. Likelihood Rating
Boston University	MA	3.69	94	72	29	9,151	9.2%	90.8%	160	23.8%	76.3%	High
Brown	RI	3.82	91	72	38	7,770	1.2%	98.8%	144	11.1%	88.9%	Very High
Case Western Reserve	OH	3.78	96	74	24	7,556	10.9%	89.1%	214	19.6%	80.4%	High
Columbia	NY	3.91	98	77	6	7,855	16.3%	83.7%	138	16.7%	83.3%	High
Creighton	NE	3.77	82	70	X	6,375	2.5%	97.5%	166	6.6%	93.4%	Very High
Dartmouth	NH	3.66	89	70	50	8,399	1.1%	98.9%	92	5.4%	94.6%	Very High
Duke	NC	3.88	97	76	12	6,951	7.8%	92.2%	121	17.4%	82.6%	High
George Washington University	DC	3.7	87	70	58	14,997	0.5%	99.5%	184	3.3%	96.7%	Very High
Georgetown	DC	3.63	85	68	44	13,149	0.5%	99.5%	203	3.4%	96.6%	Very High
Harvard	MA	3.9	97	76	1	7,613	7.6%	92.4%	165	11.5%	88.5%	Very High
Howard (HBC)	DC	3.42	53	61	94-122	9,093	0.5%	99.5%	119	5.0%	95.0%	Very High
Johns Hopkins	MD	3.81	99	76	2	6,016	6.1%	93.9%	120	12.5%	87.5%	Very High
Mayo	MN	3.92	98	76	6	7,265	6.3%	93.7%	102	5.9%	94.1%	Very High
Meharry (HBC)	TN	3.5	53	62	X	7,381	4.1%	95.9%	114	19.3%	80.7%	High

School	State	GPA										
New York University (NYU)	NY	3.93	99	77	4	8,937	15.9%	84.1%	103	21.4%	78.6%	High
Rush	IL	3.58	85	68	58	11,297	13.3%	86.7%	144	22.9%	77.1%	High
St. Louis University	MO	3.84	87	71	74	6,834	6.7%	93.3%	180	18.9%	81.1%	High
Tufts	MA	3.66	89	70	53	12,764	7.9%	92.1%	200	21.0%	79.0%	High
Tulane	LA	3.52	77	66	X	12,982	3.5%	96.5%	190	19.5%	80.5%	High
Uniformed Services (Hebert)	MD	3.64	74	66	X	3,096	6.2%	93.8%	175	8.6%	91.4%	Very High
University of Chicago	IL	3.84	97	75	17	5,683	11.9%	88.1%	90	21.1%	78.9%	High
University of Pennsylvania	PA	3.89	98	776	3	6,578	9.2%	90.8%	150	20.7%	79.3%	High
Vanderbilt	TN	3.9	98	76	18	5,982	5.1%	94.9%	97	13.4%	86.6%	Very High
Virginia Tech Carilion	VA	3.51	85	67	81	4,483	16.6%	83.4%	43	20.9%	79.1%	High
Washington University (STL)	MO	3.89	98	76	58	4,766	4.3%	95.7%	101	11.9%	88.1%	Very High
Yale	CT	3.9	98	77	15	5,776	4.3%	95.7%	104	15.4%	84.6%	Very High

Figure 4: Top Medical Schools - U.S. News and World Report, 2010-2020
—

	2010	2011	2012	2013	2014	2015	2016	2017	2018	2019	2020	Average
Harvard	1	1	1	1	1	1	1	1	1	1	1	1.0
Johns Hopkins	3	3	2	3	3	3	3	3	2	2	2	2.6
Univ. of Pennsylvania	2	2	2	4	4	5	3	5	3	3	3	3.3
Washington University – St Louis	4	4	6	6	6	6	6	7	8	8	6	6.1
UC San Francisco	4	5	5	4	4	3	3	4	5	5	6	4.4
Stanford	11	5	4	2	2	2	2	2	3	3	4	3.6
Duke	6	5	9	8	8	8	8	7	13	13	12	8.8
Yale	6	5	7	7	7	7	8	9	13	13	15	8.8
Univ. of Washington	6	9	10	12	10	10	8	12	12	12	13	10.4
Columbia	10	10	8	8	8	8	7	6	6	6	6	7.5

U Michigan	6	10	10	8	12	10	11	9	15	16	15	11.1
UCLA	11	13	13	13	12	13	14	11	6	6	6	7.5
Univ. of Chicago	13	12	10	8	11	10	11	15	18	16	17	12.8
UC San Diego	16	15	16	15	14	17	18	18	18	21	21	17.2
Univ. of Pittsburgh	14	14	15	16	17	16	16	15	13	13	14	14.8
Vanderbilt	15	15	14	14	15	14	15	14	17	16	18	17.7
Cornell	16	17	16	16	15	18	18	18	9	9	11	14.8
Mayo Clinic School of Medicine	X	26	27	27	25	27	24	20	9	9	6	20
NYU (Langone)	27	30	26	21	19	14	11	12	9	9	4	16.5
Icahn School of Medicine	18	18	18	18	19	20	21	22	18	19	20	19.2
Northwestern Univ.	18	19	18	18	18	19	17	17	20	19	18	18.3

Chapter VIII

Med School Interviews

An invitation to interview is a reason to celebrate—after all, only about fourteen percent of applicants to a given school are selected to interview, on average. However, you're now a fish in a much smaller pond with much larger fish. At a typical medical school, less than a third of interviewees are ultimately accepted (~29% average), with some schools accepting less than a quarter of their interviewees.[1,2,3,4] If you've been selected to interview at a medical school, the administration believes you are academically qualified and have demonstrated that you may fit the missions, philosophy, and curriculum of the school—at least on paper. The question is whether or not you are who you claim to be on paper, and if you can demonstrate in person that you are a good match for the school.

While your grades, scores, and essays got your foot

in the door, the competition is no longer just about who looks best on paper. Now you must mingle with medical students, admissions officers, medical school faculty, and fellow interviewees to let them see the real person behind the application. As a physician, you will have to rely on your communication skills on a regular basis to counsel patients and families, confer with colleagues, present cases, lead a team of healthcare professionals, and potentially defuse explosive situations. Part of being a good doctor is having strong interpersonal skills, so the interview is an opportunity to identify whether an applicant has traits that help or hinder their ability to get along with others.

One of the biggest myths of applying to medical school is that the interview does not matter; some applicants allege that the interview can't hurt you and that it is only used to make sure you are not psychotic. That could not be more wrong. As admissions committee members, we have seen applicants who looked excellent on paper get rejected, and we have seen sub-par applicants get accepted, all because of their performance on the interview. The interview could be remembered for how you rallied against the odds or jettisoned your chances.

The good news is much of your performance is entirely under your control. In this chapter, we will first talk about the do's and don'ts of interviewing, followed by addressing some of the most common interview questions an applicant might expect. The next chapter continues on the same thread, discussing nontraditional interviewing formats.

These include panel interviewing, hostile interviewing, and the Multiple-Mini Interview (MMI) format, which is a unique style of interviewing which is becoming increasingly more popular among American medical schools.

"Just be yourself, to a point."

Some applicants, who are aware of the importance of the interview, play an arms race with each other in an absurd battle of who can look the most sociable: students will race to the door so they can be the one to hold it open for others. Cheeks tire from smiling for hours on end. Applicants interrupt each other to well-wish a comrade who has just been called in for his one-on-one interview. For the Mother Teresas of the interviewee pool, the kindness is just a normal part of their day-to-day living. For others, the friendliness and charm are a burdensome mask worn throughout the interview day.

Ideally, you can demonstrate on interview day that you are agreeable, sociable, and communicative, and will thereby have the interpersonal skills necessary to become a good physician.

Box 18: A quantitative fact—the interview is key

Admissions officers from 113 U.S. medical schools took part in an AAMC survey, in which they rated and ranked the importance of various application data when deciding whom to invite to interview. They were also asked to do the same rankings for candidates who had already interviewed. What is clear is admissions officers around the country look for very different things when deciding whom to interview and whom to accept. The trend is that grades and scores matter more when considering who to invite to interview, while the interview itself is most important when deciding whom to ultimately accept.[5]

Ratings scale:

5 = Extremely important
4 = Very important
3 = Important
2 = Somewhat important
1 = Not important

When deciding whom to interview:

Science and math GPA: 3.7
Cumulative GPA: 3.6
MCAT total score: 3.5
Letters of recommendation: 3.4
Medical volunteering: 3.3
Personal statement: 3.2
Clinical work experience: 3.2
Nonclinical volunteering: 3.1
Leadership: 3.0

When deciding whom to accept:

Interview recommendation: 4.5
Letters of recommendation: 3.8
Science and math GPA: 3.7
Medical volunteering: 3.6
Cumulative GPA: 3.6
MCAT total score: 3.4
Personal statement: 3.4
Clinical work experience: 3.4
Nonclinical volunteering: 3.3
Leadership: 3.1

Some applicants are just able to be themselves and shine during the interviews by the virtue of who they are. These are the candidates we hope to recognize and recruit.

Box 19: Percentage of admissions officers who ask about personal characteristics during interview

In 2008, the AAMC surveyed 127 admissions officers about what they typically asked interviewees. For instance, 98% of respondents claimed they typically asked interviewees questions that assessed their motivation for a medical career. Use this list as a guide for what characteristics schools most value. (https://www.aamc.org/download/261110/data/aibvol11_no7.pdf)

Personal characteristics	%
Motivation for a medical career	98
Compassion and empathy	96
Personal maturity	92
Oral communication	91
Service orientation	89
Professionalism	88
Altruism	83
Integrity	82
Leadership	80
Intellectual curiosity	76
Teamwork	74
Cultural competence	72
Reliability and dependability	70
Self-discipline	70
Critical thinking	69
Adaptability	67
Verbal reasoning	66
Work habits	66
Persistence	65
Resilience	65
Logical reasoning	56

On the other hand, some candidates have personality flaws that may show up in the interview and doom their chances at admission. For these candidates, they cannot "just be themselves." Rather, they need to recognize their weaknesses and develop strategies to overcome or address them. We have coached the painfully shy to look the interviewer in the eye and be more engaging and interactive. We have pointed out overconfidence to many applicants and implored them to tone down their opinions and be more accepting of other people's views. For the emotionless, we teach them to simply smile and laugh more. To get a better idea of what sort of personality "red flags" may be showing up in your interviews, do practice interviews with trusted people who are willing to give you honest and sometimes harsh criticism. Better to have a friend or mentor give you negative feedback privately than to get unexpected rejection letters from the medical schools of your dreams.

What makes a great interviewee?

The best way to understand how to be a good *interviewee* is to understand the mindset of the *interviewer*. Think of your interviewer as someone bored, tired, and perhaps even jaded. They are likely physicians (though sometimes scientists, educators, and students) who may have interviewed hundreds of applicants before you. They come with their own inscrutable preferences and biases. Like most people, they may form a judgment of you within seconds of meeting you—and this first impression may be hard to overcome. They may even be nervous themselves. The experienced interviewers have likely heard every kind of response, seen every kind of interviewee, and cringe at any response that seems forced or cliché. They are looking for applicants who fit the school's missions (primary care, research, global health, rural or underserved communities, etc.), and they are looking for students who will make excellent, happy physicians. At the same time, they are looking to exclude medical students who they believe will be difficult or abrasive to work with, whom they perceive as not likely to be good with patients, or ones who are likely to drop out.

These realities create restrictions but also open up opportunities to differentiate yourself from other applicants in a positive way. The first step in getting on an interviewer's good side is simply to give them no reason to dislike you. Be enthusiastic, positive, collegial, confident, humble, and elaborative (but not long-winded). To avoid a negative first impression, show confident body language, avoid arrogant gestures, give a firm handshake, smile, be polite, dress professionally and conservatively, demonstrate good hygiene, and be punctual. To avoid clichés, take time to think about unique stories and anecdotes you can share that show originality and thoughtfulness. Give examples of activities, experiences, and interests that show you are not another cookie-cutter applicant soon to be forgotten. Prepare some talking points about your experiences that demonstrate you're a good match. Research the school, its mission, and its curriculum beforehand, and show the interviewer you've done your homework. Connect the school's qualities to yours, and explain that connection. Practice interviewing with counselors, physicians, mentors, teachers, or at the least a friend who can give honest feedback.

From our own experiences as applicants, we know it can be hard to keep all of these things in mind, so here is a streamlined checklist of essentials of what to do before interview day:

- Know your AMCAS application inside and out, especially your research and volunteer experiences. Interviewers often inquire about specific items in your application.

- Know the curriculum, mission of the school, and what they look for in their students. (This information is usually made explicit on the school's webpage.)

- Prepare anecdotes relevant to your application.

• Prepare responses to common questions (See the end of this chapter for a list of these questions).

• Anticipate giving explanations for your "red flag" attributes, including criminal offenses, low GPA, low MCAT, or a lack of research or volunteering.

• Wear a suit (and tie for gents). Dress conservatively. Don't be unkempt or purposely look outlandish. Whether you consider it superficial or not, outward appearances, cleanliness, and a well-groomed look do matter in the medical field.

• Be confident—but not arrogant. There's a fine line between the two, and the latter can be a kiss of death; for many admissions committee members, arrogance represents the #1 least desirable trait for prospective students. Advocate for yourself, show enthusiasm, and don't forget to smile.

• Be as memorable as you can be—but don't be a spectacle. Identify what makes you unique, and sell it during the interview whenever you can without being overbearing.

- Try to seem sincere. Avoid clichés, melodrama, blatant exaggerations, or nervous behavior.

- Do not memorize responses, because you will sound too scripted if you do. Instead, memorize talking points for common questions.

Open- vs. closed-file interviews

Be prepared for two styles of traditional interviewing: closed- versus open-file. In an open-file interview, the interviewer has access to your personal statement, secondary application essays, your activities list, your letters of recommendation, your GPA, and your scores. In a closed-file interview, the interviewer knows none of that until after the interview is complete and they have written up your report. Be aware some interviews may be a hybrid between closed- and open-file. Ask during the morning orientation—or even right before your interview begins—whether your interviews are closed- or open-file. If they are closed-file, it is your job to highlight your application's strengths and address head-on (or side-step) its weaknesses. Oftentimes applicants will be given the names of their interviewers days or a few hours in advance of the interview. If you have the opportunity, take the time to look up your interviewers on Google or Pubmed to learn about their background, specialty, and research interests. If you learn your interviewer is an expert in your field of research, it may be good to brush up on the details of your research projects. If your interviewer has a particular specialty you're passionate about, you can ask questions about their specialty that may end up impressing them.

Surprise! Your interview begins the moment you step on campus.

People often behave differently when they think nobody is watching. Shows like "Candid Camera," which surreptitiously film everyday people who are unaware they are under surveillance, play upon that fact. The medical school interview day can end up being like a horrible episode for interviewees who behave inappropriately.

> **Box 20: Your fellow interviewees and medical students are allies and a valuable resource**
>
> Many applicants go into their interview day viewing their fellow interviewees as competitors who must not be trusted or helped. This is a destructive mindset. In reality, your fellow interviewees represent one of your strongest resources. On your interview day, it is more likely that your fellow interviewees will be kind, sociable, and have interesting stories to tell.
>
> Most importantly, they can often give you exclusive advice. For instance, you might learn that your upcoming interviewer did not make eye contact with the applicant who interviewed before you, so you know not to be discouraged if the same interviewer avoids your gaze, too. Alternatively, a fellow interviewee may have useful insights about the strengths or weaknesses of the school that do not appear in the school's brochure.

During the interview day, there are many times when applicants are being evaluated *outside of the interview itself*, and many interviewees are unaware of that fact. The ones who are nice during the interview while acting like jerks outside of it often find themselves rejected, and they don't even realize why.

We have heard of situations where applicants behave rudely in front of medical student tour guides, admissions office secretaries, hotel concierges and janitors, and news of their behavior reaches the admissions committee. Oftentimes, medical students converse with applicants during lunch or while the interviewees wait to be called into the interview room, and the students find the applicants behaving or speaking inappropriately, and that, too, reaches the administration.

Box 21: Another hidden opportunity—med student hosts and pre-interview dinners

At most medical schools, interviewees have the option of staying overnight with a medical student host on the night before their interview, usually free of charge. Some schools also offer a student-run dinner the night before the interview. Both of these options represent an excellent opportunity to not only save money, but also allow you to meet medical students who are often more honest and forthcoming than the students who give tours and answer questions on the interview day. Oftentimes these students also give helpful hints on what the school is looking for in its applicants or how best to succeed during the interview day.

Student hosts and pre-interview dinners can have a therapeutic effect that interviewees often do not anticipate. Meeting with students and fellow interviewees before the interview day may help to calm your nerves; although sometimes you may wake up with a sore back from the couch—or floor—on which you may end up sleeping.

On a related note, most medical schools now include an interviewer who is currently a medical student at the school, and applicants often misjudge how to behave in a student interview. Many applicants feel comfortable around an interviewer their age, so they become too casual and seem disrespectful. Or the interviewee disregards the student interviewer because of the student's youth or status. In these cases, interviewees often disrespect the student or give less effort when answering questions. Little do these applicants know, the student interviewer usually has as much power as a faculty interviewer, and is often just as harsh—or harsher—when evaluating applicants.

Some schools openly disclose when students are being evaluated and when they are not. Medical student tour guides often begin the tour by stating, "Ask me anything; don't worry, I won't tell the office. You're not being judged." Other schools never disclose anything. In those instances, it's best to assume that—as long as you're on campus—you are being evaluated.

When to interview

As mentioned in chapter seven, you do not want to interview at a particular school within the first two weeks of their interview season. Admissions committee members are human beings (*really!*) and are just as susceptible to decision-making biases as anyone else. One of those biases is a "fear of missing out," meaning admissions officers are often reluctant to admit early interviewees out of fear they will admit too many applicants too early and miss out on stronger applicants who apply later in the year.

Interviewees in the first few weeks of interviews also tend to be stronger applicants than those who apply later in the admissions season, so by interviewing early, you are competing among a tougher crowd and are being judged by inordinately picky evaluators.

This does not mean you should not apply early. It just means that when you are offered an early interview, simply schedule your interview after the first two weeks that interviews begin at those schools. Most schools begin interviewing in August and September, although some schools will begin interviewing slightly before or after that interval.

You should also avoid interviewing late. If you interview too late, you will be competing for fewer spots, because many will have already been filled by applicants who interviewed earlier than you. Interviews are typically late if they occur after November. If the school practices non-rolling admissions, then your interview date cannot be considered late, because none of the seats are filled until after every interviewee has interviewed for the admissions season.

Common interview questions, responses, and analyses

Be sure to prepare for the interview day by familiarizing yourself with the most common interview questions. We've included the most commonly asked questions (and their variations), some examples of interviewee responses, and our analysis of how each response fared.

Question 1. Tell me about yourself.

Tell me about your family.

Tell me about your upbringing.

How would you describe yourself?

Answer 1 (A1): "I was born on a military base near San Diego. Being part of a military family meant I had to travel all around the world when my dad got stationed at different naval bases. I spent a lot of time in the Philippines and Japan, and I'm fluent in Tagalog. I think growing up overseas helped me gain a broader knowledge of the world and has made me more comfortable around people of different languages, cultures, and ethnicities."

Analysis: Many medical schools are affiliated with hospitals in underserved, ethnically diverse neighborhoods, so medical students will be exposed to patient populations that are economically, socially, linguistically, and culturally diverse. As a result, we like to see students who come from backgrounds that exposed them to diverse peoples and situations, because they are more likely to be comfortable and competent when treating such patients. Unusual circumstances are also simply more interesting and helps break up the monotony of meeting a litany of upper-middle class applicants who grew up in homogenous, gentrified environments. A1 is good in that it tells a story while demonstrating diversity of experience and cultural competence.

Answer 2 (A2): "My father is a pastor, and my mother is a social worker. While I was fortunate to never be in poverty, it was nonetheless always part of my life. At the dinner table my mother would discuss her work—the broken homes, the wavering social services, the cycle of poverty—and my father always played a large part in the community, organizing food drives, maintaining soup kitchens, and managing a half-way house. It made me more socially-conscious. Helping out with my dad has been a big part of my life, and for me, I want to be a doctor who specifically deals with the most marginalized communities. To me, social justice and medicine go hand-in-hand."

Analysis: It is essential that applicants demonstrate—or seem like—they are compassionate people who are interested in serving others, especially in a way that is medically relevant. While the applicant does not explain how their upbringing led them to medicine, they do a good job of explaining why serving others became important to them and how it has shaped the kind of medicine they want to do. They link how their upbringing led them to experiences that shaped their beliefs and aspirations. That demonstrates thoughtfulness and passion—and that always sets a great applicant apart from the competition.

Answer 3 (A3):"I was raised in a Dallas suburb. My mom's a nurse and my dad is an attorney. My dad was laid off for about a year when I was 12, and that was pretty rough on us; so I definitely learned what it's like to scrape by, and I think that will help me connect better with all the poor patients I'll see as a doctor."

Analysis: Be careful about overplaying your disadvantages to gain a competitive edge when applying to medical school. While the above answer may in fact accurately reflect reality for the applicant, his self-described "hardship" may not resonate as deeply compared to other applicants who grew up in poverty or truly economically disadvantaged.

Question 2. Why do you want to attend this school, specifically?

Why should we choose you over the other highly qualified candidates?

How would you contribute to the talent and diversity of our student body?

A1:"Because I want to go to a top-ranked school."

A2:"It's close to my parents and my boyfriend—he's such a hunk."

A3: "I love the weather here! I also love the city. I'm tired of the boonies."

A4:"I've tutored and have been a teacher's assistant, and I really enjoyed educating others. I'd love to continue doing that as a physician, not only as a physician teacher but also creating new medical curricula. Your school is really unique in that it offers a pathway in its curriculum to train medical students to become professional educators. The program is highly structured, well-connected, and carves out time for me to pursue my passion for education. No other school offers this great of an opportunity."

Analysis: A1, A2, and A3 may be your true reasons, but they are a little too honest. Interviewing for med school is a bit like a date with a new partner. You want to tell your partner you like them for who they are, and not for superficial reasons or mere convenience—like they have a great body(akin to A1), they live close by so you don't have to drive too far (A2), or because they have a posh studio downtown that is so much more exciting than your 2-bedroom pre-fab in the soulless suburbs (A3). A4 is a good answer because it shows you like the school for its 'personality"—in other words, its curriculum, faculty, mission, patient population, et cetera. But what makes A4 excellent is that the applicant has demonstrated—through her experiences—why she is a good fit for the school. She shows initiative and maturity by identifying her interests through activities, applying to schools that offer a special curriculum that match her interests, and explains how her passions match what the school offers. Whenever appropriate, a strong applicant explains why they are a good fit for the school to which they are applying.

> **Box 22: (True) American Horror Story: Med School Interviews—Episode 1**
>
> John, a native Californian, leaned back in his chair in an overly comfortable position. He decided to answer his interview questions with as much candor as possible, perhaps admixed with a touch of humor. So when his interviewer started their discussion with the fairly standard question, "So... why do you want to go into medicine?," John hesitated momentarily, then responded: "You see... it's always been my parents' *wet* dream that I become a doctor one day." The interviewer – although not an old-school conservative by any means – tried not to let the amazement on his face show... although effectively the interview, and John's chances of admission to that medical school, was over right then and there.

Question 3. Why medicine?

- If you couldn't become a doctor, what would you do instead?

- If you do not get into any med schools, what would you do?

- Why do you want to be a doctor? Why not get a nursing (or Ph.D., or MPH) degree instead?

Chapter 1 of this book is, essentially, the question of "Why medicine?" It may be useful to review that chapter if you want to prepare for this common—and important—interview question. Your answer should be backed up by sustained, clinical experiences. A common variant of this question is: "If you don't get into med school, what would you do?"

Applicants might assert that they would reapply or pursue some health care-related career, like nursing, clinical research or public health, which is fine (if not a little bit dull). Alternatively, you might mention a completely non-medical related field that lends insight into some aspect of your personality or character: your creative side (music, graphic design), your desire to help others (starting or working for an NPO), or your analytic ability (working for the CIA or NASA).

Question 4. Tell me about your volunteer work.

> Why did you do this volunteer activity? What did you learn?
>
> What accomplishment are you most proud of, and why?
>
> Tell me about a time you had to look through the eyes of another person.

A1: "I volunteered as a counselor at a camp for disabled children for 3 years. I was the lead counselor, and I enjoyed being in charge. It was pretty fun and we got to play a lot of games. One of the counselors and I didn't really get along—but other than that, it was good. I became good friends and a mentor to one of the disabled girls at the camp."

Analysis: *Some students think they did quite well on an interview, so they are surprised when they get rejected. Often they made a comment in passing that raised suspicions in the interviewer's mind. This is more likely to happen when a student rambles during an interview. The statement 'I enjoyed being in charge," may be (mis) interpreted as a sign that the candidate is too bossy and controlling. The offhand statement 'one of the counselors and I didn't really get along" raises questions about how personable the candidate is, if not explained in greater detail, and whether she can work well as a teammate and leader among medical school peers.*

A2: "I volunteered as a lead counselor at a summer camp for kids with cerebral palsy and quadriplegia every summer for 3 years. I'd been fortunate that nobody in my family had any serious disability, but that also meant I hadn't had much exposure to the disabled. I know it sounds cliché, but I really got to connect with a lot of the kids, especially after three years of friendship, and they are just people with problems, like everyone else— they just have a particular kind of problem that I found I could help with. One of the girls, Tina, lives close to my school. She and I became really good friends. She is quadriplegic, and now I help her after school three times a week after becoming a CNA [certified nursing assistant] for her. While she is physically challenged, her mind is so brilliant and motivated, and I am helping her get into college."

Analysis: *A much better version of A1. It supplies more details and gives a story of why the applicant volunteered and what she learned. A2 also involves going the extra mile by becoming a caregiver. This goes to show that often a better answer is not only due to style but also content. If your volunteering experience went the extra mile, don't be afraid to mention the extra effort during the interview.*

Question 5. Tell me about your research.

- Describe your research to me as if I were in middle school.

- What were you testing in your research? What were the results?

- What are the practical consequences of your research? How will your findings affect others?

A1: "I don't really remember the exact details. I did that research three years ago, and it mostly involved a fair amount of pipetting and running gels [electrophoresis]. I can email you the details later if you'd like."

Analysis: *Terrible. Always know your research for interviews. And never cast your activities in a negative light ('as grunt work").*

A2: "I did research on donepezil, an acetylcholinesterase inhibitor, and we gave it to subjects. We were seeing if it would make them better at perceptual learning. We tested that by giving them a computer task that measures perceptual learning. You see how much they learn on the drug and compare that to how much they learn with a placebo. They did better with the drug, so that means acetylcholine increases perceptual learning."

Analysis: *A better answer than A1, but not quite perfect. Your interviewer is unlikely to be familiar with your field of research, so avoid unexplained jargon ('acetylcholinesterase inhibitor", 'perceptual learning"). Remember, as a physician you will need to explain complicated technical information to your patients in a way they can understand. A2 is too technical and leaves too much unexplained.*

A3: "I've done a lot of volunteer work at an Alzheimer's clinic, and it motivated me to do research work in this field. I worked at a neuroscience lab where we studied Aricept, a drug used to treat Alzheimer's disease. Specifically, we wanted to see how Aricept improved one particular aspect of cognition. I was responsible for devising a computerized task that teaches and tests a difficult visual perception task that maps to the occipital lobe. The idea here was that Aricept increases acetylcholine in that part of the brain, perhaps enhancing how easily the brain can rewire itself there into more effective connections. We performed a randomized, double-blind, within-subjects study where 30 patients performed this computerized task while on Aricept or placebo, and found that use of Aricept did improve outcomes by 41%."

Analysis: A big improvement over A2, this answer explains the key elements of research: What is being studied, why, how, the broader implications of the results, and the applicant's specific role on the project. This is all done without being too technical. Great care was placed in explaining things in a way that a non-expert could understand. Many candidates cannot explain why they did their research or how the results could impact others. If you can explain this well, it will give you a strong advantage.

Question 6. What is your biggest weakness?

- **What is your greatest strength?**

- **What are you most worried about if you become a doctor?**

- **Tell me about a time you had to go against authority.**

A1: "Well, I admit that people get on my nerves a lot of the times... I guess I'm more of a loner by nature."

A2: "I'm just such a perfectionist. I work too hard and expect too much from myself. I end up very productive but I tire myself out!"

Analysis: *Don't be the antithesis of what a doctor should be (A1), and don't be the one-millionth phony to convert a weakness into a strength (A2), because that's lame and we can see right through it. The trick is to occupy the sweet spot between saying something too honest and negative (A1), and saying something too positive and insincere (A2).*

A3:"I like to please others, but sometimes to a fault. There are times when you need to stand up for yourself and others, especially when someone is asking you to do something unethical, disrespectful, or beyond your expertise. But in the past there were times when I didn't speak up, because I felt like if I did, then I would be confrontational, and I tried to avoid conflict when I could. This is a problem I identified many years ago and have worked on a lot over the years. In college I purposely sought out a variety of leadership experiences, and these put me in situations that required me to be more assertive. Now I feel like I am much more able to stand up for myself."

Analysis: *A3 is the compromise between A1 and A2. It gives a real weakness, but one that is not an incorrigible character flaw. It also shows good self-examination and explains how the candidate has worked on overcoming this self-identified problem. It may be useful to give a story or anecdote that demonstrates the weakness, what you learned from that episode, and how you've attempted to improve yourself. We love candidates who are humble and honest enough to show some vulnerability—just don't drop a bombshell, such as admitting you're a pedophile, drug addict or kleptomaniac.*

Box 23: (True) American Horror Story: Med School Interviews—Episode 2

Steven, a bright young Asian-American student from a top-tier college, deftly and confidently responded to one interview question after another regarding his impressive array of undergraduate activities, leadership experiences, and laboratory research. He explained articulately his motivation for wanting to enter the field of medicine, believing that it was his calling to be of service to humanity. Finally, his interviewer, sensing that the candidate was perhaps just a bit full of himself, asked him, "So, what do you think is your greatest personal weakness?" At that instant, the conversation stopped cold. Steven shifted uncomfortably in his seat, appearing confused, clearly not expecting this line of questioning. After a solid 20 to 30 seconds of silence, he stammered, "Well...I've always thought that my legs are too skinny." The interviewer shared this response with his committee afterward, all of whom had a good laugh about it and asked, "Come on...was this guy kidding?" (He wasn't.)

Question 7. Where do you see yourself and your career in 10 years?

> • **What kind of medicine do you want to practice?**
>
> • **What specialty do you like the most?**

A1: "My dad is a family doc in rural Iowa. So probably that. He already has a practice set up and everything. I could just take it over later."

Analysis: *This shows a real lack of imagination and motivation. Does this candidate even want to become a physician or are his parents pushing him?*

A2: "My dad is a family doc in rural Iowa. I've spent hundreds of hours in his family practice, and I've been lucky enough to shadow him for many of those hours— sometimes I even helped out with taking vitals and scribing the charts. Sometimes he'd make house calls too, and I liked going with him when he did that. In a small town you really get to know everyone, and that's even more true as a doctor in our town, I learned. You know the patients, their relatives know my relatives, and so on. You also know their habits and personalities, and you see how that affects their health and how you treat them as a doctor. I really liked seeing how family practice works in a rural setting, and I'd really like to follow in my dad's footsteps and continue the work he's been doing in our community. I really like that your school curriculum offers a rural medicine pathway, because I think that will help train me to be the kind of doctor I want to be."

Analysis: *In an alternate universe, the same applicant who said A1 said A2 instead, and good for him. This response cites experiences, self-reflection, and thorough explanation of why he wants to do rural family medicine. He then explains how he is a good fit for the school because of his experiences.*

A3: "I'm a huge equestrian fan. You know, horse riding and racing. In 10 years, I'd hopefully be making bank by then and could have a lot of thoroughbred horses of my own, maybe sponsor a racehorse. I'd also be riding for fun, definitely with a large country ranch of my own—you need a lot of free space to ride, obviously, if you're into horses. I definitely want an Arabian stallion of my own. Wouldn't that be cool?"

Analysis: *Don't ever mention money as a reason to become a physician. Ideally your passions are related to medicine. Being a physician should not be a means to a completely unrelated end.*

Question 8. What is the last book you read?

What is the last movie you watched?

What kind of music do you listen to?

What do you like to do for fun?

Tell me a joke.

A1: "The last book I read was called *The Windup Girl*. It's a science-fiction book that takes place maybe a century from now, in Thailand. In the future, the world is so overpopulated that, in order to feed everyone, the world relies on genetically modified crops that produce higher yields than normal crops. There are a handful of mega-corporations, more powerful than governments, and they compete with each other, inventing not only new crops but also new pathogens that target their competitors' designer crops. Currency is no longer cash, but, rather, calories. I like the story because of how it takes modern issues—like genetically modified foods, vanishing ecosystems, overpopulation, and the fear of all-powerful corporations—and uses those issues to build a plausible future and make interesting social commentary on the present by writing about a dystopian future.

Analysis: *Just don't mention 'Fifty Shades of Grey" or any other NC-17 romance novel, please. This is a very* conversational question, and, as such, we're simply gauging how well you can speak casually with others. Be elaborative and give thoughtful answers; your reading selections in some ways reflect something about who you are as a person, your character, and your interests. Speaking of which, in no way do your extracurricular choices have to be directly related to medicine; in fact, most admissions committee members prefer to see applicants with a broad and diverse range of interests. In this way, A1 is a very good answer; it highlights the applicant's intellectual curiosity and interest in social issues, both of which are admirable traits in a physician.

Box 24: (True) American Horror Story: Med School Interviews—Episode 3

Edward was an undergraduate at a renowned Ivy League college, where his father and grandfather had also attended. He was on the men's rowing team and had an excellent GPA (3.8) and MCAT score. His father was a surgeon and his mother was an accountant. He had a nice breadth of activities and a solid record. He was interviewing for the medical school where he is a current undergraduate.

An impressive performance was expected, but Edward immediately ruined his first impression through an impolite act. When he walked through the door, he met his student interviewer, age 22, sitting behind a desk. Edward was supposed to give the interviewer a packet, but instead of handing it to the interviewer, Edward tossed it sloppily on the desk, and the packet slid toward the interviewer. His interviewer immediately suspected that Edward was arrogant and entitled, and Edward's boastfulness throughout the interview only reinforced that narrative. The interviewer told the admissions committee that Edward seemed talented and able, but too disrespectful and arrogant.

The school wanted to give Edward the benefit of the doubt. "Perhaps he just felt comfortable since the interviewer was a young student," they thought. Like at Hogwarts or Oxford, the undergraduate students like Edward lived in grand houses, each with a housemaster. The housemaster was quick to politely champion Edward's qualities, describing Edward as impressive and exceptional. Then they asked the housemaster if Edward ever acted arrogant—to which the housemaster quietly admitted that Edward indeed was. Edward was rejected.

Question 9. What are the greatest challenges facing American healthcare?

> What do you think about the Affordable Care Act (Obamacare)?

A1: "There's, like, nothing wrong with the healthcare system! Last month I needed a check-up and it only cost me like ten bucks, and I only had to wait a day to see the doctor. It was tight."

A2: "Hmm, well, healthcare is really expensive for some people, right? I heard that, um, Obamacare was going to make it harder for insurance companies to get away with, um, bad stuff, you know, preying on people and kicking them to the curb when they get sick... I guess we really need to have a system like in England where healthcare is free for everyone."

Analysis: *You will be hard-pressed to find an interviewer—liberal or conservative—who finds that the current healthcare system is perfect (A1)! You must know enough about American healthcare to identify problems and suggest solutions, no matter if you or your interviewer is a Democrat or Republican. Do not overstate or oversimplify problems or solutions to healthcare, or you risk sounding naive and uninformed, as seen in A2.*

A3: "Well, I've been volunteering at a local free health clinic for two years now. In that time, I've met count-less patients who were uninsured. They suffered from some pretty serious chronic diseases, many of which could have been easily prevented if they had regular and affordable access to a family doc. Sadly, of course, they were uninsured and could not afford to pay out-of-pocket. There are millions of uninsured Americans out there, and many of their preventable illnesses get way out of hand, leading to serious medical conditions that cost much more compared to preventive treatments. We need to find a way to increase preventive medi-cal care access; if we can do that, we can cut down on healthcare spending while significantly improving—and even saving—the lives of thousands of people.

Analysis: A much better answer than in A2. In A3, the applicant linked his opinion to his experiences, identi-fied a serious problem plaguing healthcare, explained why it was a problem, and described how that problem affects the country as a whole. A3 lacks any answer of how to solve the problem, but we understand a pre-med student is unlikely to have a viable solution to solving such a complex problem.

Question 10. Do you have any questions for me?

A1: "I did some work with as a medical interpreter,

translating Spanish for the mainly Guatemalan patients at my local hospital. I'm really fascinated by doing global health research in Central America, and one of the reasons I applied to your school was due to your strong emphasis in global health. At your school, how do students get involved in global health research, especially in countries like Guatemala, El Salvador, and Panama?"

Analysis: This is a great answer. Like most other good answers, it fits in your experiences, explains how those experiences translate into interests, and then connects those interests to unique offerings that the school provides exclusively. Remember, always demonstrate how you are a good fit for a school, when you can.

A2: "Do you know where the bathroom is? I had a bunch of Gatorade today."

Analysis: Partied pretty hard last night? Sometimes applicants really do say stupid things, especially at the cathartic end of an interview. The interview isn't over until it's over, so be on your best behavior all the way to the very end.

A3: "No, I don't have any questions at all. I just really think this school is the best and, well, its reputation *obviously* speaks for itself. Thank you so much for interviewing me and I hope you have a fantastic day!"

Analysis: *Question #10 is usually the final question of the interview and is your final, lasting impression, so it is critical that you answer well. Even if your questions have truly already been answered, always have at least one question you are prepared and willing to ask. Having nothing to ask gives the impression you don't care about the school. Convince them you're a good fit for the school and ask questions about what the school offers that uniquely matches your particular interests (A1). Ask questions that can't be answered by looking on the school web page. If all else fails, these questions will work in most situations:*

- **"Why did you choose to work at this school?"**

- **"What do you like about this school?"**

- **"What makes this school stand out from the others?"**

After the Interview Day

Typically, your interviewer will write their impressions of your interview with them, and then they will send it in to the admissions committee. Many interviewers will write their interviewee report the night of your interview day or the day after. This report will be seriously considered when the admissions committee convenes to decide your admissions fate. If the interviewer is a member of the admissions committee, then they may discuss your interview performance in person during the committee meeting.

Many applicants wonder if they should send thank-you notes to their interviewers. The reality is that thank-you notes are unlikely to boost your admissions chances significantly, if at all. Send a thank-you only if you feel you are truly grateful for the interview day and want the interviewer to know how you feel. Keep it brief—no more than a few sentences—and don't suck up or sell yourself in your note. Be mindful that some schools specifically ask you *not* to contact your interviewers after the interview.

Summary

- If you are invited to interview at a medical school, your interview performance is the single-most important factor in whether you are accepted or not.

- Interviewees are judged on their performance throughout the interview day. Applicants may be rejected because they were caught being rude while on campus, even outside of the interview itself.

- There are common interview questions for which you should be prepared. Know about the Affordable Care Act ("Obamacare") and be prepared for questions on ethics and ethical dilemmas.

- Know every last detail about your application, as your interviewer may ask you specific questions about it. If you have done research, you must know your experiment thoroughly and be able to explain it to a non-expert.

- While interviewing, you must strike a fine balance between seeming too stiff, formal, and robotic, while, at the same time, not appearing too casual and disrespectful.

---

[1] https://medicine.umich.edu/medschool/education/md-program/our-community/students-faculty/admitted-class-profile

[2] https://meded.hms.harvard.edu/admissions-at-a-glance

[3] https://med.virginia.edu/admissions/about/quick-stats/

[4] https://medicine.missouri.edu/news/mu-school-medicine-introduces-class-2022-white-coat-ceremony

[5] https://www.aamc.org/download/261106/data/aibvol11_no6.pdf

Chapter IX

The Multiple (Not-So-) Mini Interviews (MMI) and Other Interview Formats

What if a sign told you there was something daunting behind a door—and that you had to open it two minutes from now? Each year, more and more medical school applicants are facing that situation on their interview day, thanks to the rise of a relatively new interviewing format called Multiple Mini Interviews (MMI). In this style of interviewing, you don't know quite what to expect until you approach the door, at which point you learn what will be inside the room. After two minutes to prepare, you enter the room to participate in a scenario. The scenario could be nearly anything. For instance, you might enter with another candidate and debate him or her on bioethics while an admissions officer listens in. Alternatively, you may encounter an actress who is playing an angry patient who refuses to vaccinate her child because a certain buxom blonde celebrity on TV said not to—and now you'll have to persuade her to accept treatment. When you're done with the first room, there are only *seven* more to go!

What is most challenging about this rollercoaster of scenarios is that they are difficult to prepare for. Medical schools that conduct MMI keep their scenarios confidential and the number of possible scenarios is too astronomical to anticipate them all. However, most of the scenarios fall into predictable categories for which you can prepare—and this chapter will review those categories in detail. We will also discuss two less common nontraditional interview formats: panel and group interviewing.

The MMI is like speed dating

What do maple syrup, Drake, and the MMI have in common? They're all exported from our ultra-polite neighbors to the north. The MMI started in 2001 at McMaster University in Canada, and since then a majority of Canadian medical schools have adopted the model.[1] As of 2020, over 45 American medical schools have followed suit with either the MMI or a hybrid—a number that is expected to grow in the coming years.

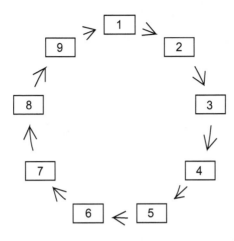

In a typical MMI format, eight applicants enter a testing area. The area consists of rooms that are typically repurposed medical examination rooms, like the ones you use when you visit your family doctor for a checkup. There are 6-10 of these rooms—or "stations"—each with a particular scenario (except for one, which is a rest station). Outside each room is a sign or sheet that briefly describes what is expected of the applicant when they enter the room. Inside the room, there is a rater—usually an interviewer—who evaluates and scores how well the applicant responded to the prompt. Candidates have two minutes to read the prompt and plan their response. When they enter the room, they have eight minutes to perform. A public address (PA) system is installed in the hallways and each room, and a voice announces when to enter and leave the rooms. The voice also warns when there are two minutes remaining for the station. Applicants who finish early often spend the remainder of their time waiting outside. Usually—but not always—there is only one applicant per station, and candidates move sequentially through the stations until they have completed the circuit of nine stations. The interviewee receives a number score for each station. These scores are computed to form a total score that represents the applicant's MMI performance.[2]

MMI: "Harder, Better, Faster, Stronger"

Most traditional med school interviews last 30 to 60 minutes—while the truth is much of that time is arguably wasted. The reality is most interviewers form strong first impressions of their interviewees within the first few minutes of the interview, and these first impressions are quite difficult to change. So, in most cases, only the very beginning of the interview really matters. By cutting the interview down to 5-8 minutes, the MMI attempts to make interviews last only as long as is useful.

Box 25: List of MMI Schools

As of January 2020, the following American medical schools conduct MMIs. Note that they may or may not also conduct traditional interviews in addition to MMI. This list is likely to expand, given the rising trend in schools adopting MMI.[3]

Albany Medical College	University of California-Riverside
California Northstate	University of California-San Diego
Central Michigan University	University of Cincinnati
Chicago Medical School at Rosalind Franklin University	University of Colorado
Duke University	University of Illinois College of Medicine
Hofstra	University of Massachusetts
Kaiser Permanente	University of Michigan
Medical College of Georgia	University of Minnesota Twin Cities
Michigan State University College of Human Medicine	University of Mississippi
New York Medical College	University of Missouri-Kansas City
New York University Long Island	University of Nevada–Reno campus
New York University	University of North Carolina
Nova Southeastern	University of South Carolina Greenville
Oregon Health and Science University (hybrid)	University of Texas – Austin
Rutgers Robert Wood Johnson Medical School	University of Toledo
San Juan Bautista	University of Utah
Stanford University	University of Vermont
SUNY Upstate	Virginia Commonwealth
TCU and UNTHS (Fort Worth, Texas)	Virginia Tech
Universidad Central Del Caribe (Puerto Rico)	Wake Forest
University of Alabama (hybrid)	Washington State
University of Arizona–Tucson and Phoenix	Wayne State
University of California-Davis	Western Michigan University
University of California-Los Angeles (hybrid)	

With shorter interviews, the MMI allows time for further interviews. In that sense, the MMI may be more efficient and may generate more data.

Another reality of traditional interviews is that interviewers often harbor particular unconscious biases and preferences that may affect how they rate the applicants they interview. If an applicant only has one or two interviewers, their chances may be doomed if their interviewer subconsciously dislikes the applicant for unfair, arbitrary, or superficial reasons. With the MMI, there are so many interviewers and judges that any one evaluator's biases are drowned out by the collective opinions of the other evaluators. In other words, the MMI may be more reliable than traditional interviewing. For those of you who studied inferential statistics, you may recall that sampled data is more valid when the sample size is larger.

The MMI is also, arguably, a better measure of interpersonal and communication skills, and it's also a superior predictor of future job performance as a doctor—according to some research.[4] By creating unique scenarios—some involving puzzles, actors, debates, and social cooperation—the MMI may be useful as a way of modeling and reflecting situations that medical students and doctors are likely to encounter in professional practice.

Because each of the MMI stations is so dynamic and unpredictable, some claim it is resistant to preparation ahead of time, so the MMI gauges a candidate's true character, skill, and ability to think on their feet rather than how well-rehearsed they are. While that is certainly true to a certain extent, *we* believe you can in fact increase your MMI score through thoughtful preparation. In particular, if you lean more toward the introverted side, you may tend not to perform as well as your extroverted counterparts in this format, according to some research. As a result, you may require extra practice and effort to overcome common "negative" behaviors, like shy or submissive body language, lack of communication, and a shortage of enthusiasm. But, in reality, everyone—even the most outgoing and confident of applicants—would benefit from familiarizing themselves ahead of time of what they might expect in this unique interviewing format.

How to make the MMI your BFF (Best Friend Forever)

The best way to prepare for the MMI is to become familiar with the various types of scenarios that may come your way. Most MMI schools employ scenarios from more than one category, so you should be prepared for each of these possibilities. We'll identify the major categories of scenarios, give some examples for each category, and describe the best strategies for each kind of situation. Then we'll round out the discussion with some general tips that can apply to any station you will encounter no matter its content.

Category 1: The mini-traditional interview

Most MMI stations will fall under the mini-traditional interview category. In this style, applicants enter a room where an interviewer is already seated. They know only your name before you enter, if that. Unlike traditional interviews, the mini-traditional interview focuses only on one interview question, with which you'll be provided two minutes before you enter the room. Outside the room, you are given paper on which you can brainstorm your response. Once inside, candidates are given eight minutes to discuss the question with the interviewer. Typically, interviewers first ask, "Do you understand the prompt?" at which point you deliver your initial impressions. Most applicants give a brief monologue answer lasting no more than 3-4 minutes. The remainder of the time is dedicated to follow-up questions from the interviewer. Some interviewers have no follow-up questions and may dismiss you early, or they may be open to further open-ended conversation. Immediately upon your exit, the interviewer rates your performance on a numerical scale.

Most of the interview prompts—but not all—are the kinds of questions you would encounter in a traditional interview or in a secondary application essay, like "What is your greatest weakness?" Or, "Tell me about a time you had to go against authority." Chapter 8 has a review of common traditional interview questions and is good review for this MMI category.

Some interview prompts present hypothetical dilemmas and problems that require you to devise a solution. Oftentimes, these problems are more than logistical—they're ethical, too. Here are some other examples of dilemmas, written in the format you're likely to encounter before you enter the station room.

'Station 6: You are a medical student shadowing a cardiologist. You and the doctor meet Mr. Evans, a 68-year-old retiree who has recently undergone replacement of his implantable cardioverter-defibrillator (ICD), a small device that detects improper heart rhythms and corrects them by sending a brief electrical shock to the heart. His previous device had been sending painful shocks at inappropriate times. After receiving his new ICD, Mr. Evans reports that he is continuing to experience shocks even from this new device, even though the tests show no shocks were ever delivered from his device. The cardiologist concludes the patient is suffering from 'phantom shocks"—in other words, shocks that only exist in the patient's mind. The cardiologist confides to you that Mr. Evans comes in every two weeks to complain about this problem, preventing the doctor from seeing other patients in the overbooked, hurried cardiology clinic. The patient is poor and uninsured, so his trips are very costly. The cardiologist decides to prescribe a placebo (sugar pill) to Mr. Evans and tells him the pill is a new drug that cures 100% of these shocks. When you are alone with Mr. Evans, he asks you if you think the pill will work. Explain to the interviewer what you would say to Mr. Evans."

delivered from his device. The cardiologist concludes the patient is suffering from 'phantom shocks"—in other words, shocks that only exist in the patient's mind. The cardiologist confides to you that Mr. Evans comes in every two weeks to complain about this problem, preventing the doctor from seeing other patients in the overbooked, hurried cardiology clinic. The patient is poor and uninsured, so his trips are very costly. The cardiologist decides to prescribe a placebo (sugar pill) to Mr. Evans and tells him the pill is a new drug that cures 100% of these shocks. When you are alone with Mr. Evans, he asks you if you think the pill will work. Explain to the interviewer what you would say to Mr. Evans."

In ethical dilemma cases, start by explaining what you believe to be the relevant issues. By showing you recognize all the sides and nuances in the situation, you show the interviewer you're perceptive, thoughtful, and not inclined to rush to judgment—no need to blurt out first thing that comes to mind, "That cardiologist is acting COMPLETELY unethically!" Impulsive responses risk alienating your interviewer from the get-go, or at the very least creating a sour first impression. Instead, framing the issues up-front allows you additional time to develop and refine your position and formulate a thoughtful response. In the example above, an applicant might note the following issues that are raised from this case: (1) Should a medical student ever give contrary advice to a patient? (2) Is the cardiologist justified to treat this patient with a placebo? (3) Is it ever ethical to lie to a patient, especially when there may be some benefit to lie? (4) Is it appropriate to weigh the needs of other patients in the clinic over the needs of Mr. Evans? You can also discuss what kinds of information is missing in the scenario that could be useful to know, like if there is an established treatment for phantom shocks of which the cardiologist is unaware.

Then you should describe the possible stances one could take, explaining why each side has its reasons. For instance, saying, "Patients trust physicians, and if a patient learned the doctor lied to them, it could seriously undermine the patient-doctor relationship and the patient may be far less likely to accept future treatment. On the other hand, lying in this case would provide tangible benefits—the patient may experience less pain, may save much-needed money by no longer going to the doctor for phantom shocks, and would allow the cardiologist to spend more time on patients who have life-threatening conditions."

Then take a stance and give reasons. If you show you understand the situation, the sides, and the pros and cons, then your stance is unlikely to offend the interviewer if he disagrees with you. For example, "I don't think it's appropriate for a medical student to contradict a physician's orders to a patient, so I would reassure the patient by telling him how much more experience the cardiologist has. But I would discuss the issue with the doctor privately and suggest he refer the patient to see a psychiatrist. Even though the placebo may provide benefit, a psychiatrist may have the appropriate expertise to address the problem more effectively, and this would be a viable treatment plan that avoids lying and undermining the trust required on both ends of the patient-doctor relationship."

Lastly, be prepared to defend your stance. You will likely have a few minutes remaining after you articulate your initial opinion. This time may be filled by questions from the interviewer about your stance. Or the interviewer may provide additional information about the scenario that could change the nature of the dilemma.

Here's another example: "*Station 3: You've been charged with planning a series of billboards in a multiethnic suburban community to increase awareness of preventative screenings for breast cancer. How would you design the campaign to maximize its effectiveness?*

This prompt is different in that it is more logistical than ethical, but the principles are the same. First, define the problem. (1) What does it mean to maximize effectiveness? Number of people who are screened? Number who identify their cancer early? (2) What are the ethnicities and cultures of the neighborhoods, and how should the billboards be tailored to each neighborhood? (3) How wealthy and educated is the community? (4) What are the financial, legal, and logistical limitations of the billboard placements? How many billboards? (5) How can the campaign take into account that some populations may have limited access to affordable healthcare, like cancer screenings?

Then present some potential solutions and critique them. You could place them in the city center where population is most dense to maximize viewership—but what if only a particular population of residents travels through the center? Or maybe you would be sure to mention that there are translator services available at the screening location. After all, you read somewhere that patients, when there is an unbridgeable language barrier, are more likely to mistrust health professionals and are less likely to adhere to their treatment plans. (Bring in outside knowledge when you can).

Category 2: Hostile interviewers

After the MMI is over, many applicants speak in hushed tones to each other about "that one station" where "the interviewer was a real jerk." Many of the applicants don't know that the interviewer was hostile by *design* (or...yes, the possibility exists that maybe he *was* just a jerk). Many stations are designed as your run-of-the-mill mini traditional interview, but perhaps at one of them the interviewer is specifically instructed to behave in a manner that unnerves the applicant. As a doctor, you will undoubtedly encounter hostile patients (not to mention potentially unpleasant staff and colleagues), so why not examine how well you cope with a hostile interviewer? You can spot a hostile interviewer by typical behaviors, like:

- A consistently blank facial expression

- Intense eye contact

- Criticism of your responses

- Rapid-fire follow-up questions

- Frequent interruption of your responses

- Bored or disinterested body language

While there is the off chance your interviewer just has a surly personality, it is more likely their role is specifically designed to unsettle you no matter the quality of your responses. You may even be evaluated on how well you cope with the stress: Do you become hostile, defensive, or nervous? Or do you act politely and resolutely despite the challenge? Once you recognize the interviewer isn't truly upset with you, the station quickly loses its bite.

Category 3: Writing tasks

There may be one station that is just like a mini-traditional interview, except there is no interviewer. Instead, there is a room with a computer you use to record your response. The same strategies apply, the only difference being written versus oral communication. We hope you're not a slow typist; but even if you are, remember that it's the quality of your response far more than the quantity. In fact, in many arenas—including medicine— brevity can be the soul of wit.

Category 4: Puzzles, games, and debates

You may have played puzzle games or social games like charades at a party—but there was probably little on the line besides bragging rights and a few laughs. Some MMI stations feel like these kinds of games, except the stakes are a bit higher. In the MMI, applicants typically encounter stations where they are tasked with solving a puzzle, playing a game, or participating in a debate, either with another applicant or with a member of the faculty. Many of these puzzles and games have "fun" restrictions, like blindfolds or forbidden words. Like any MMI station, the task is timed. At the end of the task, the rater may ask you to discern the purpose of the game or the reason for the restriction, if any. Here are some good guidelines.

- If engaged in a debate, be sure to treat the person with whom you're debating respectfully and collegially. You are not trying to crush your opponent. You can even compliment them if they make a good point.

- Med schools are looking for students who will be team players, and they desire cohesion among their students. An applicant who is ultracompetitive, abrasive, or unkind, who debates their opponent too acerbically, risks being placed in that unflattering category, "Smart...but doesn't get along well with others." When working alongside someone to achieve a common goal on a puzzle or game, be sure to be a team-player for the same reasons. It's a fine line to balance: you can't seem bossy, but you shouldn't seem passive, either. Offer suggestions rather than commands. Be encouraging and patient. If you feel you've failed a task, do not show any hint of anger, especially toward others.

Many games require you to develop strong oral communication skills. Learn how to describe objects effectively. Could you get someone to imagine, for instance, a honey dipper just by describing its physical characteristics?

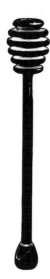

A bad description: "It's a stick—a wand!—with an...oval-ish thing at the end of the wand. The oval-thing is all sliced up."

A better description: "It's a continuously wooden rod, shaped roughly like a microphone and about the same size. At one end the rod expands to become shaped like an egg. The egg looks as if it were cross-sectionally cut into eleven evenly sliced pieces, the cuts made perpendicular to the length of the rod, then as if every other segment was removed, with the remaining segments forming an egg shape with large segmented gaps, like a hair comb."

Category 5: Role-playing situations

Some schools like to include as part of their MMI a role-playing station or two. For these tasks, a prompt describes a dilemma or situation, for which you have three minutes to prepare your response. Inside is an actor who plays one of the characters described in the prompt. Oftentimes, you are playing the role of someone else, as described by the prompt. These stations are a measure of your improvisational, problem-solving, and interpersonal skills. Here is an example of a role-play prompt:

'Station 5: You are a third-year medical student who has been doing clinical rotations in psychiatry with three other medical students. One of the students—Saul—is also a friend of yours. You notice that Saul has begun dating a female patient whom Saul met at the hospital before she was released. Enter the room and talk to Saul."

Most role-play stations will present a confrontational scenario with a character who is defensive, evasive, or hostile. Here are some helpful tips:

Discuss with the other person how his behavior hurts others and himself.

Talk about how the situation makes you feel. For instance, as a friend, perhaps you feel concerned for your friend because you care about how he has jeopardized his career.

Refrain from harsh criticism, name-calling, or describing the other person as having permanent, inherent bad qualities. For example, say, "You didn't tell the truth," rather than, "You're a liar."

Ask him to explain why he did what he did, and identify and explain any unhealthy patterns in his thinking.

Like with hostile interviewing, be sure to keep your composure. Don't lose your train of thought or your temper.

Maintain confident body language. Don't stare at your shoes. You don't need to. They're nice and polished (hopefully). Practice some scenarios with a friend and get an observer to critique your body language and tone.

Box 26: The hidden gem—the "freeform" period of the MMI

While the time to prepare (2 minutes) and the time of the station (8 minutes) is fixed, most applicants only spend 2-4 minutes actually giving their initial opinions on an interview question. The remainder—"freeform" time—presents an excellent opportunity to connect with your interviewer if he or she has no follow-up questions. You can direct the conversation to your strengths and make a great final impression.

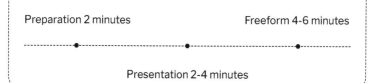

Preparation 2 minutes   Freeform 4-6 minutes

Presentation 2-4 minutes

General strategies

There are some tips that apply generally across all types of MMI stations you're bound to encounter. Here are some of the most important ones:

First impressions matter more in the MMI. With more interviewers come more first impressions. Most importantly, MMI interviews are shorter, so an applicant has less time in the MMI to overcome a poor first impression. Be sure to enter the room well-kept, polite, and give a firm handshake and a smile. Oftentimes MMI applicants end up carrying too much with them into a station, like a padfolio, sheets of paper, a pen, and a water bottle. With their hands full, they make an awkward introduction when they attempt to shake the interviewer's hand. Economize what you carry with you. Many interviewees get dry mouths, so it's fine to ask for bottled water once you're in the room (most MMI stations actually have bottled water stashed away in cupboards).

Review your written medical school application before the MMI. While most stations will not be about your extracurricular activities and aspirations, many stations end early and the interviewer will spend the extra time asking you personal questions. Take advantage of those opportunities.

Just as important as the first impression is the last—especially because MMI interviewers rate you on a number scale the moment you walk out of the room. Thank your interviewer for their participation, even if they behaved antagonistically toward you. If you respond to a stressful situation or a hostile interviewer with warmth and equanimity, this can come across as particularly impressive.

The biggest red flags are applicants who lose their composure, act abrasively, or demonstrate poor communication and interpersonal skills. The MMI is meant to test your ability to think quickly and coolly. If you have problems with that, be sure to practice some MMI-type scenarios under timed conditions with a friend, mentor, counselor, or physician.

Panel and group interviewing

In both panel and group interviewing, an applicant is placed in a room with multiple interviewers. In panel interviewing, there is only one interviewee, while in group interviewing there are multiple.

Panel interviewing

Panel interviewing allows multiple committee members to jointly and simultaneously interact with an applicant, avoiding the common scenario where the candidate wows one interviewer in the morning and completely alienates another interviewer that afternoon (often heard at meetings between admissions committee members: "Are you *sure* we were interviewing the same person?"). Undoubtedly, such a format can be a practical time-saver for institutions as well. However, recognize that the panel interview can undoubtedly be unnerving and intimidating—no matter how much the panel tries to put you at ease, the inherent nature of the format makes it inevitably stressful.

A few pointers to help you out: if you are reasonably good with names, try to make mental note of each of your panel interviewers' names and refer to them by name throughout your interview. That is sure to make a strong positive impression ("I appreciate your question,

Dr. Stevens..."). Additionally, when you answer questions, be sure to look around to give each member of the panel ample eye contact so nobody feels excluded. Addressing a group, rather than an individual, takes some practice, but it will come in handy in professional practice, when you are speaking to a patient and their family, for example, or lecturing to a larger audience.

Group interviewing

Unlike panel interviewing, admissions committees use this format to gauge how well an applicant works with peers. Interviewers will often pose the same question to each interviewee, or they will give a dilemma to which the applicants must work together and devise a solution. Just as in MMI stations that involve multiple applicants working together, the admissions officers are looking at teamwork just as much as performance in group interviews. Know your fellow interviewees' names, listen to their responses, and acknowledge their input. You may have natural leadership abilities, but there is no need to seem competitive, bossy, or arrogant with your peers to prove to them (and to the committee) you are the alpha dog or queen bee. In all likelihood, such behavior will be more detrimental than helpful to your chances. On the flip side, if you are shy, you must step up and contribute meaningfully to group conversations and the interviewers' questions.

Note that, in rare instances, some group interviewing may be done **surreptitiously**, in that the applicants are unaware they are being evaluated. For example, some schools may have a "mock classroom discussion" with a faculty member, and this session is not labeled as an "interview" on the interview day itinerary. Even in these situations, applicants are often evaluated for how they contribute to the group discussion and interact with their peers. At this point you might notice how the interview day is much more than just the interviews themselves; in truth, the interview experience begins the moment you arrive in town to the moment you leave, and your successes and failures can occur anytime in between.

Summary

- The MMI is a new kind of interviewing format that is increasingly popular among medical schools. The MMI uses "multiple mini-interviews," lasting about eight minutes each, rather than the traditional format of 30-60 minute interviews.

- It is hard to prepare for the MMI because these mini-interviews can vary greatly in what happens. Your mini-interview may be more like a short puzzle game, a debate with a fellow applicant, a role play scenario with an actor pretending to be a patient, or just a 1-on-1 short interview with a faculty member.

- Most scenarios are centered around a single question or prompt, much like the essays you fill out when applying to medical school. Thus, a good way to prepare is to review the prompts for your essays.

- No matter what the situation is, keep calm, collected, and friendly. Many MMI stations will test whether you become scared, adversarial, or immature when placed in a combative or impromptu situation.

- Be sure to make good first and final impressions, as you will meet more interviewers in an MMI than you would in a traditional format, and so your short time with each interviewer will be more influenced by their initial, fleeting impressions of you.

---

[1] http://www.medicine.usask.ca/education/medical/undergrad/prospective-students/admissions/MMI%20Fact%20Sheet.pdf

[2] http://gradschool.about.com/od/medicalinterview/a/What-Is-The-Multiple-Mini-Interview-Mmi.htm

[3] https://www.thompsonadvising.com/blog/medical-schools-using-mmi/#.X18JSmdKiU0

[4] http://www.ncbi.nlm.nih.gov/pubmed/23746161

Chapter X

The Admissions Committee

W hat goes on behind closed doors during the admission reviews process? Certainly, the goals
of any admissions committee are to be consistent and
fair—but are these goals always met? For the vast majority of schools, what goes on behind the scenes is
confidential, so applicants know relatively little of the
actions that determine their fate, which raises the
question: how transparent should the entire process be,
anyways? In this chapter, we take a look at some of the
inner workings of the admissions committee (acknowledging that no two schools have *identical* admissions
practices), from deciding who gets a secondary application to whom to invite for an interview to who, ultimately, receives an acceptance letter.

What is revealed is admissions committees comprised of individuals with—not surprisingly—major

differences in beliefs, values, and admissions philosophies, working toward assembling a class of students that best serves the interests of the medical school. Certainly, each school makes every effort to ensure the admissions process is as equitable as possible, but subjectivity and the human element invariably end up playing as important a role as test scores, grades, and pedigrees.

What does an admissions committee do?

The role of admissions committees is to make executive decisions about an applicant's admissions outcome. Committees are comprised primarily of medical school faculty (usually MDs but sometimes PhDs); at many medical schools, medical students will also be participating members whose opinions often carry equal weight to those of faculty. At a few schools, prominent members of the local community may be involved as well.

Medical schools also vary in how many different admissions committees they have, the size of each committee, and what their respective responsibilities are. Among most medical colleges, there is at least one admissions committee that evaluates applicants after their interviews to decide whether they should be rejected, waitlisted, or accepted. Many schools also have admissions committees (which are typically comprised of a subset of the above members) that meet earlier to determine which applicants receive a secondary application, and then who to invite for an interview.

Admissions committee members are tasked with evaluating, rating, and ranking applicants. Interviewees usually meet individually with at least two members of the admissions committee, who are then usually required to provide a written evaluation of the applicant prior to the admissions committee meeting. These reports are based on the interview as well as careful review of all their application materials.

The interviewer is then responsible for presenting the applicant for discussion and evaluation during the committee meeting—acting as their primary advocate, if you will. As such, you should treat your interview as an opportunity to give your interviewer all the compelling reasons they need to make their best case for your candidacy when you are discussed at a committee meeting.

How are admissions committees structured?

Many medical schools interview over a thousand applicants and, as such, cannot evaluate every interviewee using just a single admissions committee. Therefore, these schools use multiple admissions "subcommittees" with each interviewee being discussed in only one of these subcommittees. This is usually a random process, although at some schools, applicants may be sorted by specific categories. At one school, for example, all underrepresented minority (URM) applicants are reviewed by a special admissions subcommittee, staffed by URM faculty, whose sole focus is evaluating URM candidates. At another school, applicants are sorted by their undergraduate institution. For instance, subcommittee A might evaluate the interviewees from Stanford University, Rutgers University, Grinnell College, and a handful of other schools, while subcommittee B may handle those hailing from Amherst College, UNC-Chapel Hill, Tulane University, etc.; how these groupings are decided may be arbitrary, based on some historic rationale, or rooted in other tangible factors.

These subcommittees may be populated specifically by faculty and medical students who are alumni of these same institutions, which allows some in-depth knowledge of how to interpret applicants' files. While reviewing an applicant's file, a reviewer may wonder: Did they take classes that were challenging or easy? Which on-campus extracurricular activities did they list that were meaningful and substantive vs. simply social clubs that padded their résumés? In the above examples, there is more direct comparison with your similar peer group: URM applicants are evaluated relative to other URM candidates, while students from a given college are compared to those who attended the same institution. Of course, each prospective medical student from within these groups then still has to be considered in the context of the broader applicant pool.

These subcommittees will then report their recommendations to a central committee, typically comprised of the admissions dean and other senior experienced admissions officers, which takes all the subcommittees' findings into consideration to come up with a final adjudication. In deciding whom to admit, the central committee seeks to ensure its student body has a balanced composition of talent, achievement, ethnicity, and experience that reflects the values and mission of the medical school. For instance, if the committee notices that the class is overrepresented by high-MCAT super-geniuses and underrepresented by candidates who excel in other ways (e.g., a varsity athlete, an accomplished musician, or a poor applicant who overcame adversity), it may choose to revise the rank-order lists provided by the various subcommittees.

One reality of having multiple subcommittees is that one subcommittee may be harsher than another and thus rate its interviewees lower than another more generous subcommittee. Because an applicant cannot control which subcommittee evaluates him or her, there is a degree of arbitrariness to this stage of the admissions process—a "luck-of-the-draw" phenomenon that also occurs when the applicant is assigned his or her interviewers, who may or may not have similar values, backgrounds, or beliefs as the interviewee. A central committee may be able to mitigate some of these effects by adjusting for the differences in selectivity among the subcommittees—for instance, by boosting the ratings for applicants belonging to a harsh subcommittee, or by admitting an equal number of applicants from each subcommittee.

What goes on during an admissions committee meeting?

The activities of an admissions committee meeting depend, in part, on the role of that particular committee.

Committees that grant secondary applications or interview invitations

At some schools, there are admissions committees that determine which applicants are given a secondary application and/or whether they are invited to interview. These "gatekeeper" committees are typically smaller and use metrics that are easy to review and tabulate—like MCAT scores, ethnicity, GPAs, and even the prestige of the undergraduate institution attended. This system is used because there are too many applicants and not enough resources to review each one meticulously at this early stage of the admissions process.

Some schools use a point-based system, by which applicants are assigned points according to multiple criteria. This may include receiving a certain number of points based on extraordinary academic achievement, coming from a disadvantaged background or geographically underrepresented region of the country, or attending a particularly prestigious undergraduate institution. Applicants who exceed a certain point threshold will be given an interview invitation automatically, while those who fall below it may receive more scrutiny from the gatekeeper committee. Again, this committee may be overridden by an executive committee or the dean of admissions, who may choose to invite an applicant to interview despite the candidate's receiving poor marks from the gatekeeper committee. This may be due to any number of reasons: the applicant having personal connections to the school, for example (such as being the child of a faculty member), or some other unique angle that the committee may be unaware of.

Committees that interview and rate applicants

The admissions committee (or subcommittees) responsible for determining the fate of interviewed applicants will convene on a regular basis throughout the interview season, typically monthly or twice-monthly.

During those sessions, anywhere from 10 to 30 candidates are discussed. As described previously, each candidate is presented to the committee by one of their interviewer(s) who is in the best position to describe the candidate's strengths (and weaknesses) based on their personal interactions with the applicant during the interview, and careful review of the application file. Other members of the admissions committee are also expected to have reviewed the interviewee's application and record prior to the meeting, which may include the interviewers' written evaluations.

After the applicant is presented to the committee, the floor is then open to discussion regarding the applicant's suitability for admission. The topics of conversation revolve around grades, MCAT scores, disciplinary actions, bad or incomplete grades, letters of recommendation, and extracurricular records. Stellar applicants—like a trilingual varsity athlete with a near-perfect MCAT score, or a formerly homeless applicant who started a nonprofit foundation in his or her underserved community—may require relatively little discussion; their acceptance is almost certainly assured, and the committee may spend more time strategizing how to recruit that superstar to their school.

On the other end of the spectrum, a subpar applicant who came across as uninspired during his or her interview may also not require much time before he or she is summarily placed in the "Reject" pile (yes, some of these applicants somehow make it through the interview stage). The bulk of discussion (and debate) revolves around that large middle tier of candidates who sit below the top 10% but above the bottom 10%. These individuals have a number of positive attributes, a strong but not sensational record, and perhaps one or two points of concern in their application file. While much of the discussion is structured and formal, it often is interspersed with committee members sharing humorous or disastrous interview stories or opining on the merits, or ridiculousness, of an applicant's listed hobbies and activities.

What is debated when evaluating applicants?

The most heated debates stem from core differences of opinion among members of the admissions committee. The most fundamental differences center on which traits, qualities, and activities should be most highly valued when assessing applicants. With anywhere from 10-25 people on each committee, there is invariably going to be a wide range of opinions about who the school should accept and why. The following represent categories for which committee members may hold very different priorities when considering and ranking applicants:

- Extraordinary intelligence and academic performance

  Many admissions committee members feel the quintessential quality of a good physician is a superior intellect. Stellar MCAT scores, near-perfect GPAs, exclusive academic awards and achievements, and productive participation in scientific research are viewed as signs the applicant is exceptionally smart, driven, and can thrive in the intellectually rigorous world of medicine. Particularly for research-intensive schools, academic superstars are highly coveted as they represent the ones who are most likely to effectively contribute to the medical research ongoing at the school and—perhaps, one day—pioneer new and groundbreaking efforts. This in turn would enhance the reputation of the school. Committee members who prioritize intelligence above all may be more willing to overlook a less well-balanced portfolio—for example, fewer extracurricular or volunteer activities—and, conversely, are less willing to accept applicants who may embody other important traits for a physician (e.g., compassion, kindness) but just can't cut it intellectually.

- Compassion and humanitarianism

  Other admissions committee members hold the philosophy that while becoming a physician may require reasonable mental and analytic skills, it's not rocket science—hence, as long as a candidate meets a certain threshold of intellectual capacity, that is good enough for admittance. What they are searching for are candidates with a heart of gold—ones who demonstrate compassion and a desire to serve others. These characteristics are the most essential traits to becoming an effective physician—not an overwhelming intellect. Hence, applicants with less than stellar MCAT scores or grades may be given leniency if their extracurricular record demonstrates a sustained and consistent passion for serving others, particularly the disenfranchised. For liberal-leaning and service-oriented schools, an altruistic record may be more highly valued among a greater proportion of the admissions committee.

- "Seems like a nice, all-around good person"

  - Some committee members enjoy applicants who are just solid, well-rounded, good citizens. Their application files are strong, even if no one activity sets them apart in spectacular fashion. They interview well and give their interviewers a good gut feeling. The common refrain here is, "I'd love this guy (or gal) to be my physician."

- Overcame physical or socioeconomic adversity

  - As reflected by America's deep political divide, there exists, not surprisingly, fundamental differences in opinion amongst admissions committee members regarding how much weight a candidate's background should play in deciding his admissions fate. Some faculty love hearing "rags-to-riches" stories of someone who overcame poverty, homelessness, or was the first in his or her family to graduate high school or college. These committee members advocate to admit such applicants even if their scores and grades are somewhat below average, arguing that these individuals are that much more deserving because they had to overcome significant obstacles to get to where they are. On the flip side, some admissions members feel uncomfortable showing any sort of preferences on this basis, especially if this keeps out other candidates who have a stronger record of achievement or academic ability. As one might imagine, these philosophical differences can lead to lively debates during committee meetings, with the touch-point being a B+ student from a single-parent home who worked his way through state college and had little time for other outside activities. Do they deserve a chance, even if it comes at the expense of an A student from Yale who came from relative privilege?

- Academic pedigree

    Some committee members prefer applicants who have attended a prestigious undergraduate institution, and are easily swayed by name recognition (whether they are willing to admit it or not). In their eyes, the reputation of their medical school looks that much better to external observers when they can tout that a quarter of the incoming class graduated from an Ivy League school. On the other hand, other admissions faculty may have an active distaste for what they perceive as elitist institutions, and they make special effort to "level the playing field," so to speak.

- Connections to the school

    Candidates applying to the same school where they received their bachelor's degree are often viewed favorably. Similarly, applicants who have a strong relationship with prominent faculty—especially medical faculty—tend to be given preference by most members within the admissions committee. At most institutions, applicants who are sons or daughters of alumni or medical faculty are given careful consideration; their application is viewed in the most favorable light.

Leadership

Medical schools are always on the lookout for applicants who have a history of leadership, in the hopes that these candidates will continue to be leaders when they become physicians. These movers and shakers will, in turn, enhance the prestige of the medical school where they received their degree. Some admissions committee members are particularly impressed when an applicant has demonstrated initiative in creating a new organization, has risen through the ranks of an existing impactful group, or has worked tirelessly within an institution to make creative or meaningful positive change. An applicant may be highly valued if he or she, for instance, led a project to create a smartphone application for diabetics, even if their grades or interview performance were not among the very best.

Medical students on the admissions committee

It is commonplace for medical students to not only interview applicants, but to also serve on the admissions committee.

Box 27: An example of an interviewer's written evaluation of an interviewee, presented at the committee meeting

When I first started talking to H.Z., she was a bit robotic. She spoke quickly and in monotone. She seemed focused on getting her many messages across. It was difficult to follow her because she skipped around different topics. I was worried for her. However, as she got more relaxed, I finally got a chance to get to know this interesting and pleasant young woman.

H.Z. is applying to the MSTP (medical scientist training). She had done a great deal of research already, and this was clearly the focus of her application. She started doing research in high school. This was facilitated by her dad who is a pharmacist working at GlaxoSmithKline. Her research was in mental diseases.

At her college, H.Z. continued to spend the bulk of her extra time in research. She first worked in an animal lab looking for mouse models of schizophrenia. She did 10 hours per week and full time during the summer. She left that lab because she wanted more patient exposure and also because of some interpersonal issue that we did not get into. She then started working with a neurologist doing research on aphasia. In this position, she had her own research projects. She did a lot of cognitive and language testing of patients. She did most the interviews herself. She estimates dedicating six hours per week in the project during school. She expects to be doing similar types of neurologic research when she gets to medical school. When I probed H.Z. about her research findings, she was able to describe her projects adequately. However, I was not overwhelmed by the depth of her explanations.

I asked H.Z. if she was better suited for a PhD since it appeared to me that her main focus was research. She explained that when she was working with mice, she did feel somewhat unsatisfied dealing with only animals. This was one reason she moved to human research with the neurologist. Apparently, she found doing clinical research in human subjects more satisfying. Based on this experience and also the advice of her research mentor, she made the decision to pursue an MD PhD. She also mentioned the advantage to her family of having some expenses covered in the MSTP program. It seems like she comes from a modest background. Her mother is a physical therapist.

The one thing H.Z. would change about her school is to make it more social. She explains that everyone is too focused on schoolwork and academic pursuits. H.Z. assured me that she doesn't just study and do research; she is on the swim team (which is a club sport at her university) and is a member of the Circle K Club. Circle K is a service organization. She described quite vividly how they work with inner-city elementary schools. She seemed genuinely involved in this organization and dedicated to their activities.

Overall, I found H.Z. to be pleasant, intelligent, and focused. She was interesting to talk to, but not terribly interesting. I liked her, but I was not overwhelmed.

Although these students are typically younger and less experienced than their faculty counterparts on the committee, at many schools they may have the same responsibilities, privileges, and degree of influence. For example, if a medical student voices a negative opinion about an applicant, that person may be rejected, even if he or she was otherwise well-regarded by the rest of the admissions committee. Many applicants may be unaware of the amount of influence a student interviewer can wield, and may be surprised when they find out they were rejected after a less than stellar interview with the student interviewer.

How committees make their final decisions

After an interviewee has been discussed at the committee meeting, the members give their final assessment of the candidate before moving on to the next applicant. This may be done by assigning the applicant an overall rating, whether it be on a scale from one to ten, a grade of A through F, or a simple Accept/Waitlist/Deny. The scores or ratings among all the committee members are tabulated to form a composite score for each applicant, which allows a rank order of that pool. If there are multiple admissions subcommittees working in parallel, the list of their applicants, along with their final scores, are given to the central committee, which creates a master rank-order list, perhaps weighing certain subcommittees' scores more or less depending on how harshly or leniently they tend to grade. As noted above, this committee also has the authority to bump individuals up or down on the list based on special factors as well as to ensure a balanced incoming class. This list is a dynamic one, with candidates moving higher or lower on the list as the interview season progresses, and dependent in part on whether admissions are on a rolling basis or not. In the end, the top students from that list will be offered admission, the next group will be placed on a waitlist, and the bottom tier will be rejected outright.

Box 28: "We have too many of those applicants."

One reality of the admissions process is that some admissions committee members have their own biases and preferences, often related to their own background. A member who was in the rowing team in college may have a special affinity for applicants who were also on that team at his alma mater, or another faculty member may feel disdain for applicants who appear different from the students she remembered from when she was a student.

For instance, at one top-5 school, an applicant was a Vietnamese immigrant from a disadvantaged family who worked part-time to support her family. She had a great MCAT and an excellent GPA from an elite school in the Northeast. She was an accomplished violinist. In all, she was a breath of fresh air compared to many of the other applicants, who came from a more advantaged upbringing. After her interviewer gave her a positive recommendation, an older admissions committee member interjected and said, "We get a lot of those Asians, and with better numbers."

Rather than compare an applicant against the body of applicants as a whole, some admissions faculty prefer to compare an applicant against other applicants who appear to have similar qualities—for instance, comparing Asian applicants against other Asian applicants. This is clearly not fair, but it happens.

Box 29: Applicants with personal connections

While the admissions faculty tries its hardest to be impartial, there is occasionally a handful of applicants who manage to gain admission because of their strong connections to the medical school.

For instance, one applicant to a prestigious program was the son of a prominent and influential physician at that medical school. He came from a small liberal-arts college in the Northeast with a 3.4 GPA and an MCAT in the 80th percentile. The average admitted applicant for the school, at the time, had a score at the 95th percentile and a 3.8 GPA. He was on the rowing team in college, but otherwise had a mediocre list of extracurricular activities. Although the subcommittee liked applicants with an affiliation to the school, it was decided the candidate didn't measure up. The subcommittee recommended rejecting the applicant.

For most any candidate, this decision would have been final. Rarely would an executive committee overrule such a decision. Nonetheless, the applicant somehow appeared on the list of accepted students by the time school began for first-year students. Connections help.

Summary

- Admissions committees make key decisions about an applicant's outcome throughout the admissions process, including whether they will receive a secondary application, an interview invitation, and finally an acceptance to the school or not.

- Committees are comprised of MD faculty but may also include PhDs, medical students, and even members of the community.

- Your interviewer is your advocate who presents your application file to the others at admissions committee meetings, but all committee members have a say in rating you.

- Medical students are often full members of the admissions committee, and their opinions can be influential.

- There is some arbitrariness to the process: not only who your interviewers are and what traits they prize as most valuable, but also which admissions subcommittee ends up discussing your application file, as each may have its own unique biases. Recognize that some of these aspects of the admissions process are simply out of your hands.

Chapter XI

Handling Invitations, Waitlists, Acceptances, and Rejections

E very year, thousands of applicants find thick envelopes, thin envelopes, or high-priority emails
in their physical and virtual inboxes, each bearing
heart-fluttering or soul-crushing news regarding final admissions decisions from medical schools. But
these letters are hardly the final chapter to a lengthy
saga; rather, they are often just the beginning to an entirely new story. The high-fives, drunken celebrations,
mass text messages, and Instagram posts that follow
the acceptance merely precede tough choices about
which school to ultimately attend. Some applicants will
linger in admissions purgatory, their names placed on
waitlists of indeterminate length, hoping they will be
accepted only weeks—or days—before medical school
begins. Over half of all applicants will face the despair of

unanimous rejection, but for many their failure will reveal weaknesses which are overcome when they successfully reapply.

In this chapter, we will review how you should handle the three major final decision outcomes: rejection, waitlist, and acceptance. We will describe these outcomes in terms of how and when they are released, keeping in mind that applicants typically receive decisions from multiple schools at different times, often while they are still interviewing and waiting to hear back from other schools. Of special importance is how to get accepted off a waitlist and how to have a successful reapplication in the event you are rejected everywhere. We will also discuss how to pick which school to attend if you have the pleasant dilemma of dealing with multiple acceptance offers.

The admissions timeline

While excitement and disappointment are the emotions that often accompany the news of the final decision, the prevailing emotion up until that point is one of uncertainty, because applicants usually wait weeks and months after interviewing to hear final word of their status. One can never predict exactly when news will be released, but there are some general patterns to the admissions process.

Here is the rough timeline by which medical schools

interview, deliberate, and release their admissions decisions. Note that this timeline does not apply to DO or Texas MD schools. As of 2020:

Late May – Year 1: Applications begin

An applicant can submit the AMCAS application to medical schools after AMCAS verifies the applicant's transcript (after May 28th).

Early July – Year 1: Submissions begin

Medical schools begin to send out secondary applications to students who have submitted their verified AMCAS application. Some schools send all applicants a secondary application, while a few send out secondary applications selectively. For these schools, applicants may receive rejections before the secondary application stage.

Late July, August, September – Year 1: Interviewing begins

Medical schools begin reviewing students who have completed their secondary applications. Students may be rejected outright, invited for an interview, or sometimes simply placed on hold. Schools will then interview students beginning at this stage and continuing into February, March, or even as late as June of the following year. Interviewed students are ranked for final decisions purposes, but acceptances cannot be given out yet.

October to November– Year 1: Admissions decisions begin; interviews hit peak

Medical schools are permitted to send acceptances beginning mid-October. High-ranked interviewees are offered acceptances by mail, email, or phone. Middle-ranked interviewees may be placed on hold or waitlisted. Low-ranked interviewees may be placed on the end of a waitlist or rejected. At schools with **non-rolling admissions**, ranking occurs only after all students have been interviewed, and all students will hear decisions regarding their fate at the same time at end of the admissions process. Conversely, for schools with **rolling admissions**, ranking occurs in batches throughout the year, and students receive final decisions at various points throughout the admissions cycle.

December, Year 1 – January, Year 2: Interview season continues

At many schools, interviewing has passed the halfway mark. At schools with rolling admissions, the later year, and students receive final decisions at various points throughout the admissions cycle.

December, Year 1 – January, Year 2: Interview season continues

At many schools, interviewing has passed the half-way mark. At schools with rolling admissions, the later an applicant is considered, the worse his chances are, because there are fewer available seats as the cycle progresses. At this time of year, accepted and waitlisted candidates begin filing financial aid applications to the federal government (FAFSA) in anticipation of financial aid offers that schools release to accepted applicants in March, April, and June of Year 2.

February to March – Year 2: Interview season is winding down

Most medical schools begin to finish their interview invitations and interviews. At non-rolling schools, admissions committees are busily ranking *all* of their applicants so final decisions can be released in one large, comprehensive batch. By February, some rolling admissions schools will be interviewing students even though there are few or no available seats left. In these cases, desirable interviewees are, at best, placed on the waitlist.

March – Year 2: Final decision flood

Most non-rolling schools release all their admissions decisions at this point in the season. At some of these schools, all admitted students are notified in one batch, then all waitlisted and rejected students are notified a day or two later in another batch. By March 15th, each medical school must send out enough acceptances to fill its expected number of incoming students. A few schools may still be conducting interviews up through this period and even later.

April to June – Year 2: Applicants decide where to attend

Schools begin courting applicants to whom they sent acceptance offers. Many schools hold "second look" events in which prospective students revisit the school, talk with current medical students, and evaluate whether the school is a good fit for them. Schools release financial aid offers to prospective students, including scholarships, grants, and loans.

April 30 – Year 2: Applicant decision deadline

Applicants must hold only one acceptance offer by this date. Those who hold multiple acceptance offers after this date may have their offer rescinded by the school. Applicants do not have to drop their waitlist positions. Waitlist positions are valid until the school begins instruction.[1]

April 30 to end of June – Year 2: Waitlist recruitment is at maximum

By the April 30th deadline, students with multiple acceptances are forced to abandon multiple offers, thereby freeing up a great number of positions at medical schools across the country. Medical schools tend to send more acceptance offers than they have space for, in anticipation that many accepted students will enroll at other schools. Since so many students enroll elsewhere, most medical schools will still have empty seats despite the fact they overbooked. To fill those empty seats, schools will recruit off the waitlist. The bulk of waitlist movement occurs during this time interval.[2]

August to September – Year 2: Medical school begins; final waitlist admissions offers sent

Most medical schools begin instruction. Once instruction begins, the school is very unlikely to accept any students off the waitlist. Some schools will make a few last-minute offers to waitlisted students weeks or even days before school begins.

What to do if *waiting for an interview invitation*

Most rejected applicants are rejected before the interview stage; therefore, receiving an interview invitation is the largest admissions hurdle to surmount. Invitations are almost always given out by email, although a few schools post this information on their application website that students must log onto. Schools rarely invite applicants strictly in the order in which they received the candidates' applications—the selection process is usually too complicated for that to happen. If you are still waiting even though you know someone who applied after you has been invited to interview, that is not necessarily bad news.

> **Box 30: "In the area" emails**
>
> Applicants often receive interview invitations at schools located far from where they live. Traveling to interview at these schools can be quite costly, and medical colleges understand this and try to help by accepting "in the area" emails.
>
> If a student receives an interview invitation at one school, A, and has also applied to a nearby school, B, then they can email school B to say they have an interview at school A and are "in the area." School B will then expedite the interview invitation review process so it can—perhaps—send an invitation to the applicant quickly, allowing them to interview at schools A and B in the same trip. This can save an applicant from the expense of two separate trips, and offer the additional bonus of allowing an applicant to interview at school B sooner than he or she otherwise would have.

Nonetheless, if you have heard nothing by the time

the school's interviewing season is winding down, it is reasonable to send an email or letter to the admissions office. Remember that, at rolling schools, the later you interview, the worse your chances are. If you have any *significant* updates—like a new semester of good grades, a research publication or presentation, or a new volunteering activity you've been actively involved in (for more than a few weeks)—feel free to mention those. Even if you have no updates, you can always write a letter explaining how you are still very interested in the school. At best, it will encourage an admissions officer to rereview your application, and at worst it will neither help nor harm you. That being said, only send letters when appropriate, and keep them brief. Don't pester the office with repeated inquiries or it may come back to bite you.

What to do if *waiting for a final decision*

At the end of your interview day at a medical school, it is likely that someone will inform you when the school anticipates releasing its decisions. If it is a non-rolling school, then all interviewees will find out their admissions fate on the same date, usually in late February or early March. If it is a rolling school, then your decision date depends on how the school processes its applicants;

sometimes, interviewees (especially highly desirable ones) may hear back as early as one to two weeks after interviewing. The school may contact you by phone, email, mail, or any combination thereof, although phone calls are almost always acceptances. Remember, if you learn that another interviewee has received an acceptance, and you have yet to hear anything, this is not necessarily bad news, even if the other applicant interviewed *after* you did. Admissions committees rank their interviewees using algorithms that are complex and not necessarily linear; so, for the sake of your mental health, do not jump to conclusions. Wait for the news to come out rather than speculate needlessly on your chances.

Box 31: Importance of med school prestige in obtaining residency positions

For the 2018 NRMP Program Director Survey, 1,233 residency program directors were asked to cite factors they used to select which med school graduates to interview for their residency programs and rate each of the importance of each of these factors from 1 (not important) to 5 (very important).

These were the results:
(https://www.nrmp.org/wp-content/uploads/2018/07/NRMP-2018-Program-Director-Survey-for-WWW.pdf)

Selection criterion	% Citing Factor	Avg. Rating (1-5)
USMLE Step 1 score	94%	4.1
Letter of Rec in specialty	86%	4.2
USMLE Step 2 score	80%	4.0
Grades in required clerkships	76%	4.1
Any failed USMLE attempt	70%	4.5
Class rank	70%	3.9
Grades in clerkship in desired specialty	67%	4.3
Membership in Alpha Omega Alpha (AΩA)	60%	3.9
USMLE Step 2 Clinical Skills pass	56%	4.2
Medical school reputation	**50%**	**3.8**
Demonstrated involvement/ interest in research	41%	3.7

And, just as with waiting for an interview invitation, it can help to send an update (ideally no more than one) to the admissions committee highlighting notable new accomplishments, and/or a new letter of recommendation from someone whom you did not include in your original packet. These may be added to your file and possibly tip the scales in your favor if your application is a close call. It is also possible, however, that the admission committee discussing your application has already convened and hence this additional information may not see light of day; either way, no harm, no foul.

What to do if *accepted*

Congratulations! There is no limit to the number of acceptances you may hold until April 30th, when holding multiple acceptances may result in the rescission of your offers (i.e., after that time you should hold only one acceptance). However, you are allowed to remain on an unlimited number of waitlists. Your position on the waitlist is generally invalidated when your waitlisted school begins classes, or if you begin classes at another school.

If you have multiple acceptances, you have one of the nicest dilemmas you'll ever have to face: which medical school do I attend? The reality is that any American medical school will give you an excellent education, so the simplest answer is that you should choose the school that you think is the best fit for you personally and will best prepare you for your envisioned career. Of course, there are a number of important factors that many applicants need to take into consideration when comparing medical schools. Some of the biggest are:

1 ---- Cost of attendance (COA)

The median COA for 4-year medical schools was $256,000 for in-state public schools and $338,000 for private schools in 2020, according to the AAMC.[3]

The COA can vary significantly depending on grants, scholarships, and the school itself.

In-state residents typically have subsidized tuition at their state schools.

We recommend waiting on financial aid and scholarship information before declining an acceptance offer, unless you're absolutely sure you do not want to attend that school no matter the cost. Many schools hold off on grant, loan, and scholarship awards until May.

2 ---- Prestige

In a 2018 national survey of 1,333 residency program directors, medical school reputation was rated 3.8 out of 5 of important considerations that directors use when evaluating which medical school graduates to invite to interview. By comparison, earning good grades in clerkships and a high USMLE Step 1 score were both rated above 4. See Box 31 for more.

That being said, whether openly stated or not, most if not all residency programs do find it desirable to fill their slots with candidates from the very best medical schools they can (e.g., based on national rankings and reputation), as this lends additional credibility and status to their programs.

Prestige is highly linked to research funding, which may be important for applicants who aspire to do high-level research or become physician scientists.

Prestigious medical schools typically are associated with top-tier residency programs. Students at these schools have a better opportunity to work and interact with faculty at the school's affiliated hospitals and "make their mark." This can make the difference when applying to residency at those hospitals, when in-house candidates may have a distinct advantage as known commodities.

3 ---- Curriculum

A growing trend among medical schools is the replacement of a letter-grade system to a pass-or-fail system (P/F) in the first two years (the pre-clinical years) and sometimes also the last two years (the clinical or clerkship years). This reduces competition among medical students and, thereby, greatly reduces stress during medical school.

- Many schools are shifting away from lecture-based learning to team-based or problem-based learning, also known as "flipped classrooms," in which students become the teachers, and the instructor becomes a listener who guides the students as they teach each other. This can be a blessing or a curse, depending on your preferred learning style. Maybe you love learning from your peers in this way and thrive in such a learning environment. Or maybe you think that a $50K annual tuition warrants receiving more direct instruction from nationally renowned faculty members who are leading experts in their fields.

- Some schools adopt more clinical exposure during the pre-clinical years, allowing students to interact with patients well before their clinical rotations in years 3-4.

- Many schools now record and "podcast" their lectures online, allowing students greater convenience during their first two years of school. Conversely, other schools have mandatory attendance and dress codes.

4 ---- Location

- Attending the same medical school as the place you hope to do your residency may offer a competitive advantage, as noted above. However, more broadly, choosing a medical school geographically based on where you'd ultimately like to end up is probably not necessary and cuts both ways (positively and negatively). While residency directors may be more familiar with local schools and hence have a tendency to accept greater numbers of applicants from those schools, they also value geographic diversity and may specifically want to look beyond their local region and state to fill their programs.

- Choosing a medical school based on your love of the city it's situated in and your anticipated quality of life (it's near a beach! I can go surfing!) may be a legitimate factor in your decision-making process, but it probably shouldn't be the leading consideration. Certainly, proximity to family—especially if you help with the care of a family member or are responsible for other aspects of family life—does matter and represents a legitimate basis on which to help decide where you want to be spending the next four (or more) years.

5 ---- Other considerations

- Does the school have any special programs that suit

anticipated quality of life (it's near a beach! I can go surfing!) may be a legitimate factor in your decision-making process, but it probably shouldn't be the leading consideration. Certainly, proximity to family—especially if you help with the care of a family member or are responsible for other aspects of family life—does matter and represents a legitimate basis on which to help decide where you want to be spending the next four (or more) years.

5 ---- Other considerations

- Does the school have any special programs that suit the kind of career you envision for yourself? This can include dual degrees, rural medicine programs, global health opportunities, and more.

- Has the school ever been at risk of losing its accreditation?

- What kind of assistance, mentors, counseling, and support do students get?

- What is the student culture like? Do students here seem happy and satisfied? Do they complain about the school? Do they seem especially stressed?

- Will I need a car? How safe and how expensive is it to live here?

- Does the school have a good match list? This shows where graduates went on to do their residency.

> **Box 32: "Second look" events**
>
> Many schools invite accepted applicants to have a "second look" at the school before they decide on whether or not to attend the school. These events, typically held in April, are an excellent way for applicants to get a feel for whether the school is a good fit for them. During this time, applicants can attend classes and, most importantly, get a good idea of whom their classmates would be—should they attend—since a substantial portion of the attendees will ultimately decide to matriculate. It is also a valuable time to speak with current medical students and ask about the school. The impression you get of the school may be quite different and more accurate than the one you formed on the interview day.

What to do if *placed on the waitlist ("waitlisted")*

It is normal for waitlisted applicants to feel disappointed, angry, anxious, confused—and, sometimes, even relieved. The waitlist can mean good news, bad news, or no news, depending on the school, your perspective, and, most importantly, what actions you take after you've been waitlisted.

The significance of the waitlist depends on how the waitlisting school processes its interviewees. It actually may be an encouraging sign at schools where the waitlist is reserved for the few, strong applicants who were just below the cut and have an excellent chance of eventually being accepted. At some schools, up to half of the student body is composed of applicants who were accepted off the waitlist. On the other hand, the waitlist may keep you in perpetual limbo, especially for schools that tend to waitlist a significant proportion of the applicants they do not accept outright.

Although schools may have different practices in this regard, it is still hard to predict what an applicant's chances are of getting off a waitlist. There are sometimes significant year-to-year fluctuations in the number of applicants who are accepted off the waitlist. This is often due to the fact that the size of the waitlist depends on the number of accepted applicants who withdraw their position in the class in order to attend another school. Medical schools overbook their class in anticipation of this fact, and sometimes they overbook too much—such that they have few or no spots left to offer to applicants who were placed on the waitlist. Other times, schools overbook too little, and an unusually high number of applicants are accepted off the waitlist.

The waitlist is formed in different ways, depending on whether the school practices rolling or non-rolling admissions. At schools with non-rolling admissions, waitlists are given out at the same time all other decisions are made, which is around March. At schools with rolling admissions, the waitlist forms during the interviewing cycle. In batches throughout the year, interviewees are accepted, waitlisted, or rejected. At some schools, interviewed applicants are not waitlisted outright and are, instead, placed on hold or are deferred. In a deferral, candidates are in a state of limbo, as the admissions committee is unsure of whether to accept the candidate or not. Each time the committee convenes to decide upon interviewed applicants, the deferred candidate is compared to the newest batch of interviewed applicants. The committee will either accept the deferred candidate or defer them again until they consider the next batch. This process continues until the end of the year, usually around March, when all candidates who remain deferred are placed on the waitlist.

Applicants may or may not be made aware they are deferred. Some schools will practice both deferral and waitlisting simultaneously.

Most schools rank the students on their waitlist, and, if they pull students from the list, they start from the top and work their way down. Waitlisted students may move up the list if they demonstrate they are likely to attend should they be accepted. Some schools will let students know their rank on the list. If you know you are low on the list, it is up to you to decide whether you think it is worth the effort to lobby to move up the list. In theory, students may be pulled off the waitlist at any time, but, in practice, they tend to be pulled off in May and June, because on April 30th, students may only hold one acceptance, so as students drop their acceptances, waitlist positions begin to open up. Schools may continue to accept students off their waitlist in smaller numbers all the way until school begins, typically in August.

If you are waitlisted or deferred, the first question to ask yourself is just how interested you are in attending the school. If you are genuinely excited about the possibility, you should properly demonstrate your enthusiasm by letting them know you are very likely to accept an offer, should they grant you one. You should also share new, significant updates about what you have been doing since you last were in contact with them. A new job, recent good grades, published research, or a new volunteering activity are all good things to mention.

It is important you convey these messages in the right way. First, find out how the school prefers to hear from you. Some schools have an online application page specifically meant for updates and correspondences. Others prefer you to email the admissions office. Either way, write a letter that combines your interest in the school with any new updates, if any. There are two major flavors of these kinds of letters. The first is the **letter of interest**, which is a letter that explains the school remains "one of your top choices" and that you are still very interested in attending. The second is a **letter of intent**, which explains the school is your *top* choice and that you would *definitely* attend their school if they offered you a position, *no matter what*. The latter can carry more weight, but, obviously, you should only send it to one school. You may also include a letter of recommendation from someone (ideally a faculty member or physician) who can speak in some detail on a new activity or accomplishment you wish to highlight. Keep your update brief and simple, and sound enthusiastic rather than desperate. Only send in a single letter, and don't email the dean or your interviewer directly. That's too pushy.

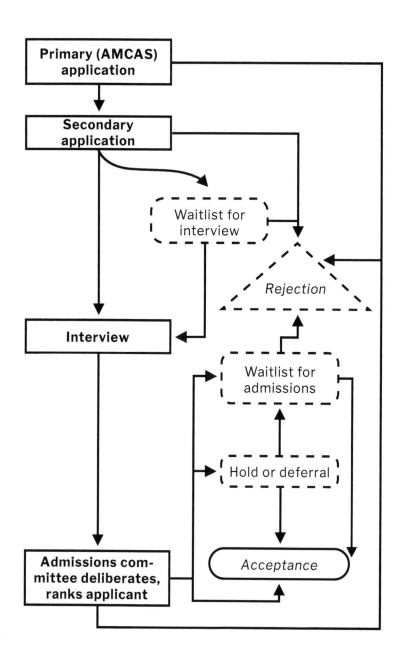

What to do if *rejected at a particular school*

Rejections can come at any time during the admissions process, from the moment you submit your primary AMCAS application all the way to the day the school begins its classes. Most schools notify by status update on the online application portal, or by mail and email. A few schools "silently reject," meaning a rejection is implied if you do not hear from them by the time their classes begin.

There is not much you can do if you are rejected. At some schools, you can file an appeal, but this is very unlikely to succeed. The only situation in which it may work is if someone very influential writes an appeal on your behalf. An example would be a senator or a highly regarded professor at the school to which you are appealing. Even then, the odds are slim.

If you've been rejected from your dream school and have been accepted elsewhere, it can be tough to decide whether to attend the less-desired school or wait another year, improve your application, and reapply in hopes of getting into the school of your dreams. In general, reapplying is a risky gamble—there are no guarantees in the admissions process. We know of students who gave up acceptances at lower tier schools so they could reapply, only to find themselves with no acceptances a year later. Although there are occasional exceptions, most who apply again to schools that previously reject-ed them are rejected again. In addition, some admissions officers may see it as a red flag that you were accept-ed at a medical school yet decided to reapply anyway. If you are concerned that the school you've been ac-cepted to is too low-ranked to allow you to pursue your goals, you may be mistaken, especially if you work hard and perform well at whatever place you end up. If you are still adamant about reapplying, see the next section.

What to do if rejected and how to reapply

The biggest reason applicants reapply is because they were rejected from every school to which they ap-plied. During the AMCAS application cycle of 2019, 41% of all students who applied were accepted to medical school, meaning that 59% were rejected everywhere they applied, according to the AAMC.[4] If you fall into this category, there could be a number of reasons why:

- Applied too late to medical schools

  - Schools with rolling admissions fill up their seats throughout the year, so applicants who apply late are competing for fewer available seats. Applicants have the best shot when they apply as soon as they can, by submitting their AMCAS application at the end of May and filling out secondary applications promptly.

Applied to the wrong medical schools

Some applicants apply only to schools that are too much of a reach (for example, an applicant with a 508 MCAT score who only applies to schools with a 518 MCAT average). GPA can be a similar issue. While it doesn't hurt to aim high, it may be time to realign your expectations with reality.

Some schools have an exclusive or strong preference for in-state applicants—usually public state schools. Applicants who apply from out of state have a much lower chance of being accepted at these schools.

Some schools strongly prefer students who wish to practice rural or family medicine; other schools strongly prefer students who are interested in research and academic medicine. If you do not fit the school's preferred profile, then your chances are slim.

Most schools make their preferences clear on their school website. Do your research before applying.

Applied to too few medical schools

Most schools have an acceptance rate well below 10%.5 By applying to only a handful of schools, your risk of not being accepted to any of them goes up. It is not uncommon for applicants nowadays to apply to 40+ schools, and you should apply to just as many, if not more, your second time around.

- You have one or more "red flags" in your application, such as:

- Poor grades, poor MCAT score

- One or more bad letters of recommendation

- Weak secondary essays and personal statement

- An institutional action or criminal record

- Bad interviewing skills

- Not enough volunteering or extracurricular activities

To have success the next time you reapply, you need to identify the weak spots that got you rejected. Some red flags are easier to discover than others. Some easy ones to spot are poor MCAT and GPA, coupled with choosing schools that accept students with much higher grades and scores. Felonies, plagiarism, and cheating offenses are other obvious major obstacles. But some debilitating attributes may be harder to spot. For example, letters of recommendation are usually unread by the applicant and may contain negative remarks. Because letters of recommendation are typically strong among most candidates, a poor or lukewarm letter looks especially bad (see Chapter 6 on Letters of Recommendation). Some applicants are also poor interviewees and are unaware of their bad performance. A clue you're a bad interviewee is if you received many interviews yet were ultimately rejected by all of the schools at which you interviewed. In these cases, your application was strong and consistently earned you interview invitations, but your interview itself sunk your chances. Some schools will let you know why you were rejected. Did you come across as disinterested? Arrogant? Superficial? It doesn't hurt to call the admissions office and ask. Counselors and advisors may also be useful resources in identifying what went wrong with your failed application.

To have any chance of a successful reapplication, you *must* reapply with new, substantial changes that ameliorate your previous deficits. This may take more than a year, depending on what is wrong with your application. Here are some common problems with solutions:

- Poor MCATs

  - Identify whether your learning style, study time, study support, and study materials were sufficient the last time you prepared for the MCAT. Change your strategy to maximize your re-take score.

  - Any subsection with a score below 125 is often a red flag. Concentrate your studying in these particular areas of weakness.

  - Consider applying to a Doctor of Osteopathy (DO) medical school. They tend to accept medical students with lower scores.

Poor GPA

Post-baccalaureate programs are tailored toward pre-med students looking to repair their GPA. Consider taking additional classes to boost your GPA and to prove you have a new, strong track record.

A special masters program (SMP) is a 1-2 year program that allows students to take graduate-level science courses, often alongside medical students. These programs are often used by pre-med students with low grades or MCAT scores to prove they can handle the rigor of medical school, provided they earn good grades (i.e., nearly all A's).

Both post-baccalaureate and SMP programs sometimes offer linkages to affiliated medical schools, meaning admissions to medical school is guaranteed provided the applicant earns a good GPA in the program and does well on the MCAT.

DO schools allow for grade replacement, meaning you can retake a class and the new grade will replace your old one. This allows for significant GPA improvement, should you apply to DO schools.

Felonies, institutional actions in college

Oftentimes, the longer these offenses are behind you, the better your chances are.

Exceptional volunteering and altruism may make a difference in cleaning up your image.

For example, if you received a DUI (driving under the influence), then becoming a speaker on the danger of drunk driving to high school or college-aged kids may show how you have learned from your mistakes.

For many schools, serious criminal offenses can never be overcome and your chances at medical school admission will remain poor.

Common examples: unlawful sexual behavior, domestic violence, assault, child abuse, sexual assault, prostitution, public lewdness or exposure, sale of narcotics and controlled substances

- Poor letter of recommendation

Consider whether you had any letter writers whom you did not know well, or may have had any reason to dislike you. Do not ask them for a letter again, and find letter writers who can speak about you on a personal level and you are sure will be able to focus on your positive attributes and accomplishments.

- Poor interviewing (also refer to Chapter 8 on interviewing)

Seek out a trusted friend, mentor, counselor, adviser, or physician to do a mock interview, and ask them for honest feedback. It is best to find a physician since they will surely have done medical school interviews in the past either as an interviewer or interviewee.

Some students find it helpful to film themselves during a mock interview to discover any negative body language or behaviors.

Consider whether you answered these key prompts well. Include them in mock interviews and get feedback:

Why medicine?
Why our school?
Tell me about yourself.

Applying too late, to too few schools, and/or only to highly selective of schools

See Chapter 7 for more details

If you do reapply, it is essential you address head-on in your personal statement and secondary essays the weaknesses you had in the past and how you have overcome these weaknesses. In that sense, you can frame your reapplication as an example of perseverance, which, in turn, has strengthened your character. Every year, many people reapply to medical school and find themselves significantly more successful.

Summary

After you apply to a medical school, waiting for their final decision on your application can be difficult. Schools may not be transparent on how or when they decide on your application.

Medical schools tend to have a set schedule of when

they read applications, invite applicants to interview, and decide whom to accept. Knowing this schedule—and where you fit into it—may help you keep track of how your application is being processed throughout the year.

Some schools accept students throughout the year ("rolling admissions"), while other schools accept all their students at the end ("non-rolling"). For the former, the later you interview, the less your chances of admission are, because you are competing for a smaller number of available seats.

Getting an interview is generally harder than getting accepted. In other words, most applicants are rejected before receiving an interview invitation. If you have not received an invitation to interview by the time their interview season is closing, send the admissions office an update letter, if you have a significant achievement to share.

If you are waitlisted after an interview and still want to attend, send a letter voicing your interest to attend, along with any significant updates. Acceptances off the waitlist tend to happen in mid-May, so sending a letter a 2-3 weeks prior may be the best time, although this may vary from school to school.

If you are not accepted anywhere, consider why your application was considered weak. It could be your GPA, MCAT, criminal record, disciplinary action, a bad letter of recommendation, poor interviews, or perhaps you applied too late. If you do reapply, your application must be much stronger, as few applicants are ever accepted after applying more than twice.

---

[1] https://www.aamc.org/students/applying/

[2] https://www.aamc.org/students/applying/recommendations/370684/trafficrules-applicants.html

[3] https://www.usnews.com/education/best-graduate-schools/the-short-list-grad-school/articles/most-expensive-private-medical-schools#:~:text=Paying%20for%20four%20years%20of,for%20the%20class%20of%202020.

[4] https://aamc-orange.global.ssl.fastly.net/production/media/filer_public/1e/7e/1e7ea68f-94da-4667-8123-c04c5ce34e41/2019_amcas_infographic.pdf

[5] http://www.doctorpremed.com/medical-school-acceptance-rates.html

Chapter XII

Minority, Older, and Disadvantaged Applicants

There is more to an applicant than their academic performance, the school they attended, or even what extracurricular activities they pursued—and admissions faculty acknowledge and value that fact. Many applicants must overcome significant challenges to attain a level of achievement comparable to that of their peers. These candidates have *traveled a greater distance* to be where they are now, and that counts for something in the admissions process. This may include a single mom who worked a job during college to support herself and her child, a gay applicant who faced significant discrimination in a prejudicial community, or a Latino candidate who is the first in his community to apply for graduate school.

In addition to looking for candidates who have over-come adversity, admissions faculty value applicants who they believe have the potential and desire to be-come leaders in communities that are traditionally un-derserved or impoverished. It has been shown that pa-tients feel more comfortable receiving treatment from physicians who share the same ethnic and cultural iden-tity and values, so many medical schools seek to train physicians who plan to serve and give back to the com-munities from which they came, and where there are few doctors that match the patients' backgrounds.

Medical students from unusual or marginalized backgrounds also bring new and diverse perspectives and experiences that they can share with their peers. This makes the student body more eclectic, which many medical schools highly value. In that sense, many schools also seek out well-rounded, older applicants who can contribute their storied history of experiences and previous careers to enrich the student body.

Figure 1: Acceptance by race, 2018-2020 (aggregated), AAMC

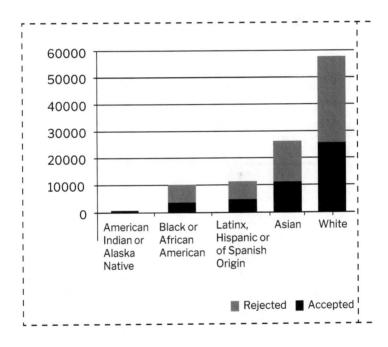

Figure 2: Under- and over-represented ethnicities in medicine (AAMC '19-'20, US Census 2019)

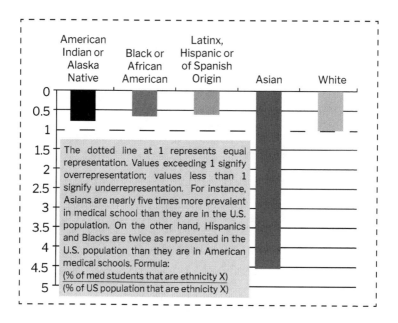

In this chapter, we will review how admissions committee members commonly perceive minority, older (30+ years old), and economically disadvantaged applicants. We will also discuss how these identities should shape your application to medical school, if applicable.

Minority applicants

The corridors of most medical schools are lined with yearbook portraits of previous graduating classes. Inspect these portraits, and you will see that in decades past nearly all the students fit a single profile—white and male. Since that time, admissions committees have attempted to construct a student body that more closely resembles the demographics of the people whom those students will serve as physicians.

While men and women are about equally represented in medical schools today, certain minority groups are considered "**underrepresented in medicine**" (**URM**), including those of African, Native American, and Hispanic or Latinx descent. For instance, only 8.8% of accepted applicants to medical school in 2019 were Black, according to the AAMC, while Blacks composed 13.4% of the nation's population, as reported by the 2019 US Census.[1,2] Conversely, Asians have been considered a minority group heavily "**overrepresented in medicine**" (**ORM**), composing 24.8% of accepted applicants while being only 5.9% of the U.S. population.[1,2] Many medical schools recruit URM applicants to help bring about equal representation in the field of medicine.

There are three core reasons medical schools seek out URM applicants:

1 ---- The belief that URM students will contribute and share their unique experiences and perspectives when interacting with fellow medical students who do not have the same background. This enriches the student body and enhances the students' cultural competency, which is their ability to interact effectively with patients who have a different set of experiences, beliefs, and expectations from themselves.

2 ---- URM students will become physicians who will act as leaders within their communities to promote positive social change.

3 ---- URM students will become physicians who can better understand and treat patients who share the same ethnic, linguistic, or cultural background as the doctor. Some studies show that patients are more likely to follow medical advice, report their symptoms more accurately, and feel more cared for when their physician shares the same background as they do.

Because medical schools place such a high value on URM applicants, admissions faculty may be willing to admit URM candidates who have test scores and grades that are below the school's total average. Thus, if you are a URM applicant, you should not necessarily be deterred from applying to schools that have higher average scores and grades. The following graphs describe success rate at getting into medical school from 2010-2012 by ethnicity.

Box 33: URM-focused medical schools and student programs

There are some programs within medical schools that have a mission to train students to serve specific underserved and ethnic communities—there are even a few medical schools in which this mission applies to every medical student. These programs and schools are often less selective with respect to MCAT and GPA scores, but they are more selective when it comes to recruiting applicants who have competence, experience, and passion for under-served and underrepresented patient communities.

Many medical schools house special programs that focus on disadvantaged or underrepresented ethnic communities. The three historically black medical schools—Meharry, Morehouse, and Howard—especially value involvement with the African American community. Here are examples of some other programs:

Latinx/Hispanic

- PRIME-LC, UC Irvine
- Latinx Health Pathway, University of Rochester

Urban Underserved

- PRIME-US, UC San Francisco
- Area Health Education Centers Program, Saint Louis University
- Urban Medicine Program, University of Illinois at Chicago

Underserved

- Sam W. Ho Health Justice Scholars Program, Tufts University
- Charles R. Drew/UCLA Medical Education Program

Some medical schools highly value accepting URM applicants on the basis of improving diversity in their school and the field of medicine. For these schools, it is a significant advantage for you to simply identify yourself as a URM applicant when you select the race(s) you most identify with on your primary AMCAS application.

Note that most schools also request a photographed portrait of you on their school-specific secondary application. Obviously, applicants who misrepresent their ethnicity can jeopardize their odds of admission.

Stronger yet are URM applicants who have faced significant obstacles in life due to racial prejudice, or candidates who have been leaders in improving their community. The AMCAS personal statement and secondary essay prompts are excellent outlets to share stories of obstacles you may have faced. The AMCAS activities list is ideal for listing leadership and volunteering activities that have served your community. Examples include being a peer mentor, a community organizer, a big brother to an inner-city child, or president of your local Black pre-medical society in college.

Figure 3: Percentage accepted into a medical school by MCAT, 2010-2012 (AAMC), N=80,375

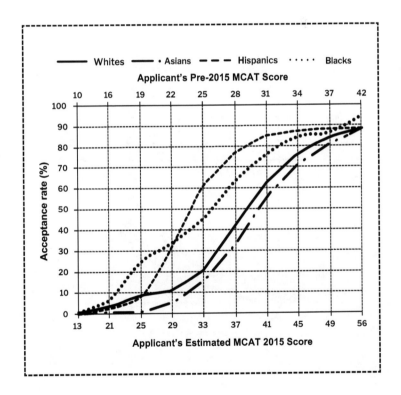

Figure 4: Percentage accepted into a medical school by GPA, 2010-2012 (AAMC), N=80,375

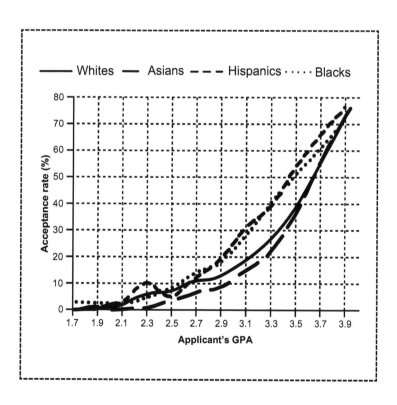

Some URM applicants come from families that are economically and educationally disadvantaged, and these candidates have overcome significant obstacles to be where they are now. While there is often a link between URM applicants and economic disadvantage, there are some who come from affluent backgrounds and have lived an educationally and economically privileged life; for instance, they attended elite private schools, grew up in gated communities, and were raised by parents who were, for instance, high-powered attorneys or surgeons. Admissions committees may still value the ethnic background of such applicants, and hence it is still worthwhile to share community involvement and stories of overcoming racial prejudices, if relevant. However, as is true no matter what your ethnicity or background, it is important that you not overstate or fabricate obstacles that you did not truly encounter.

> **Box 34: LGBTQ+ applicants**
>
> Some applicants of the LGBTQ+ community wonder if they should mention their identity in their applications or during medical school interviews. The answer is that it depends on (1) your personal level of comfort and the degree to which your sexuality defines you, and (2) a recognition of external factors that may influence your admission, either positively or negatively.
>
> Most medical schools openly recruit and value LGBTQ+ applicants, like Columbia, Emory, and the University of Pennsylvania. Some religious and conservative medical schools, however, may not.
>
> If your sexual identity was a significant obstacle—due to, for instance, growing up in an extremely prejudicial and hostile environment—it may be worth mentioning. Additionally, if you advocated for or led within the LGBTQ+ community or have a passion for LGBTQ+-related health and are applying for medical schools that specialize in furthering those goals, then bring that up as well. However, it may be preferable to focus on other aspects of your accomplishments and identity in your application essays and interviews if you did not experience LGBTQ+-related struggles and do not have particular activities or health-related goals associated with the LGBTQ+ community.

Socioeconomically disadvantaged applicants

We strongly admire medical school candidates who have overcome socioeconomic and educational hurdles, no matter what their ethnicity is. In such circumstances, an applicant's achievements are magnified because they were that much more challenging to attain. On the same note, their academic and extracurricular shortcomings can be explained by more pressing concerns—like working a night job to pay for food, struggling to find a stable place to live, or sacrificing a significant amount of time to care for an ailing relative. We also commend applicants who come from rural or disadvantaged communities or were raised by parents who never graduated from high school or attended college, because those applicants show great initiative by, for example, being the first to attend or graduate from college and apply to medical school, essentially stepping out into unchartered territory.

Admitting economically disadvantaged applicants also adds diversity to medical schools. According to a 2017 study, around 12% of first-year medical students came from families whose income was in the lowest 40 percent—while around 73% of accepted students came from the top 40 percent.[3] Medical school students with humble origins may bring different experiences, values, and viewpoints that can enrich the student body. There are a few ways to describe your disadvantages to the admissions faculty. There is a checkbox on the primary application, which you can mark if you want to be considered as "disadvantaged." You can also describe your struggles in your AMCAS personal statement and how these struggles may have shaped various aspects of your application, such as less-than-stellar grades during your freshman year transition or during stretches when you had to work long hours to keep up with tuition payments. Many schools offer specific essay prompts, asking applicants to write down any significant challenges they faced.

The AAMC developed a "socioeconomic status disadvantaged indicator" in 2014, which is used to give a standardized classification of socioeconomic status to all of its applicants. The indicator specifies the extent to which an applicant is disadvantaged, ranging from EO-1 (most disadvantaged) to EO-5 (least). It bases its classification on the parents' level of educational attainment and whether their labor is professional or manual. Interestingly, the AAMC does not consider family income when computing a candidate's socioeconomic status indicator. Admissions committees also evaluate whether applicants have received Pell Grants or whether the applicant indicated if they lived in a disadvantaged or rural county.

Many applicants worry about marking down that they are socioeconomically disadvantaged under the misconception that a school is less likely to recruit poor applicants because they are less likely to be able to afford tuition.

Box 35: Profile of LQ, a disadvantaged applicant

LQ grew up in a poor, rural community in the Midwest. Most of the residents—including her parents—worked at a large chemical manufacturing plant. Neither of her parents went to college, and her mother dropped out of high school when she became pregnant. Both her parents held manual labor jobs processing chemicals. LQ was the second eldest of her five siblings.

LQ worked a part-time job through high school to help her family of eight make ends meet. Nonetheless, she excelled in sports and academics and was the first to attend her state university, where she received some financial assistance.

She majored in biochemistry and was doing well up to her sophomore year. Her GPA declined from a 4.0 to a 2.8 after she had to commute back and forth from home and college to act as a caregiver for her father. He had begun to suffer from a chronic and debilitating spinal condition.

Despite this, she managed to continue her studies and her final GPA was a 3.35. She also won an award for research she conducted with faculty at her university on how a certain chemical may be responsible for a severe allergic form of contact dermatitis. She designed this study after noticing many people in her hometown had dermatitis, likely due to chemicals they encountered at the local chemical plant. During vacations and on the weekends, she also volunteered at a local free health clinic that served those in the community who were uninsured and could not otherwise afford to see a doctor.

LQ applied to medical schools that had an emphasis on rural medicine and family practice since she was interested in returning as a physician and tending to people in her community. She was admitted to almost every school to which she applied. While in medical school, she continued her skin-related research and became fascinated by dermatology, which she eventually specialized in. She is now a dermatologist in her local community, treating many of the work-related skin conditions she studied as an undergraduate researcher.

Box 36: How the AAMC determines level of socioeconomic disadvantage

The parents' educational attainment and their jobs are used to determine an applicant's level of disadvantage—not their family salary. EO-1 is considered the higher of the two disadvantage indicators. In 2013, 20% of applicants were EO-1 and 7.8% were EO-2 according to the AAMC.
(https://www.aamc.org/students/services/332852/aftersub-shared3.8.html)

	Executive, managerial, professional position	Service, clerical, skilled, and unskilled labor
Doctorate or professional degree	Not disadvantaged	Disadvantaged: EO-2
Master's degree	Not disadvantaged	Disadvantaged: EO-2
Bachelor's degree	Not disadvantaged	Disadvantaged: EO-2
Less than bachelor's	Disadvantaged: EO-1	Disadvantaged: EO-1

Virtually every medical school in the United States practices need-blind admissions, meaning applicants' ability to pay is never counted against them. In fact, medical schools—especially top-tier private ones—offer generous need-based scholarships, grants, and low-interest loans to lower-, middle-, and, sometimes, even upper-middle class students. Another mistake many disadvantaged students may make is that they feel too sheepish or hesitant to discuss their social and economic hardships. To these applicants, we implore:

Take pride in what you have accomplished, especially when the circumstances of your achievement were difficult. This only increases your chances of acceptance.

Disabled applicants

A common fallacy is that disabled students cannot become doctors. Many schools have an official list of "technical standards" for medical students, which require students to possess aptitude in observation, communication, sensory and motor coordination and function, cognitive ability, and behavioral and social skills. However, some schools are willing to modify these rules—or help students meet these rules—under certain circumstances.

Medical schools have admitted applicants bound to wheelchairs, with lost limbs, and with dwarfism, for example. In 2005, Tim Cordes—who is blind—made history when he graduated near the top of his class with a medical degree from the University of Wisconsin-Madison. He is now a psychiatrist.

However, disabled applicants should be sure to recognize that their training and future careers will be different and more difficult compared to their more able-bodied peers. If you are disabled, contact medical schools before applying and ask if and how well your condition will be accommodated, because schools will vary in such policies. Also be aware that, depending on the nature of your disability, you may be prevented from practicing certain specialties that require specific motor functions you are unable to perform.

If you have suffered a debilitating condition, it is likely to have represented a significant obstacle or transformative experience—and you can certainly mention this in your essays and personal statement when applying to medical school. But beware that some of the worst essays and personal statements we've read have come from applicants who overplay their illnesses. Don't write an entire personal statement on your struggles with early male pattern baldness, for example.

Also be aware that mental disorders may represent an equal, or sometimes even greater, red flag in your application. While honesty is always the best policy, writing about your history of mood disorders or schizophrenia may raise concerns amongst admissions committee members regarding your suitability to withstand the rigor of medical school and a future medical career. This may be true even if your disorder is well-controlled and represents a battle you have strived to overcome.

Box 37: Profile of MM, an older applicant

MM is a 33-year-old applicant. He earned a Bachelor of Science degree in biomedical engineering and helped design pacemakers for people with abnormal heart rhythms. During his job, he often worked with cardiologists and monitored the surgical insertion and removal of pacemakers.

While MM enjoyed engineering, he found that his favorite part of the job was seeing how his finished products were installed in real people. He liked the concreteness of seeing how physicians improved the lives of patients on a one-on-one basis. He asked one of his closest colleagues, a cardiologist, if he could see more. The doctor agreed to let MM shadow her. He found he enjoyed other aspects of the job besides the pacemakers—he liked how the doctor would check and follow up on patients at her clinic. He liked seeing how the pacemakers she installed led to improved health, mood, and outlook in the patients who came back for a return visit.

MM decided he wanted a career where he could mix his love of devices, engineering, science, and newfound appreciation for patient care. He took a few additional science courses at a local post-baccalaureate program to fulfill his pre-med requirements, took the MCAT, and applied for an MD-PhD dual-degree program.

When he got into such a program, MM furthered his studies and research in electrical engineering through his PhD studies, while learning medicine through his MD studies. MM is now a professor of cardiac electrophysiology and does clinical research on pacemakers while helping his patients attain healthy heart rhythms.

Older applicants and career changers

Traditionally, students begin medical school right after graduating from college. However, many schools are increasingly seeking non-traditional applicants who have taken one or more years off before matriculation. For example, 68% of the 2019 entering class of

University of Pennsylvania's medical school were so-called nontraditional.[4]

A sizeable minority of these non-traditional students are much older than the average first year student. Each year, medical schools receive a modest number of applications from candidates who are *over 30 years old*. Many of these older applicants have made significant progress in another career, such as academia, engineering, finance, law, or education. Some have experience in the medical field as nurses, health care administrators, or biomedical researchers. A great number of these applicants have tremendous success getting into medical school based on their maturity and breadth and depth of experiences, and the path by which they ultimately chose medicine forms a better narrative.

It is important to dispel the myth that older applicants are summarily dismissed by admissions officers because of the applicants' age. For the most part, age only becomes a negative factor among some admissions faculty after the age of 40. This is because the length and cost of medical training means a 45-year-old first-year medical student would become a fully trained physician at age 53 or later. Because of the high cost and significant resources involved in training a physician, some consider it financially impractical and socially irresponsible to train someone who will only be able to practice medicine for a relatively short amount of time before retirement. There may also be some doubt as to how well a candidate in their 40s and 50s can handle the typical rigors of residency training. All these caveats notwithstanding, each applicant's unique circumstances and impetus for entering medicine at a significantly older age will be considered on a case-by-case basis, and if you are an extremely strong candidate, you should not be discouraged from applying.

Admissions committee members find it both fascinating and worrisome when an older applicant switches their career to medicine from some other unrelated field. On one hand, having a well-developed career adds a level of experience and uniqueness that is unparalleled in younger, more traditional applicants and adds diversity to the student body. On the other hand, it raises the question of someone's fickleness and level of commitment to a chosen field (if you are abandoning business or law, who's to say you won't do the same to medicine?). It may appear that you've had a mid-life crisis and are using medicine as an escape route or a road to riches and prestige.

To dispel that worry if you are an older applicant, it is especially critical for you to prove that you have thoroughly examined whether medicine is a good fit, and that you are doing it for the right reasons. You should have *sustained* exposure to the field of medicine prior to applying, whether shadowing physicians, volunteering at hospitals, or working as a scribe or EMT for more than a few months (none of which may be easy if you already have a full-time career!). This may not be an issue if you already working in a medically-oriented field (e.g., as a nurse, technician, or health care administrator). Your application essays will be your best opportunity to articulate why you are leaving your previous career and why you plan to enter medicine instead. These essays should ideally offer a compelling narrative of how you arrived at making a career switch and what, specifically, draws you to medicine. The reasons cannot be wealth or influence, or that you are simply burnt-out from your current line of work. For a review of "good reasons to be a doctor," refer to Chapter 1.

Most older applicants will not have taken all of the pre-medical classes required for medical school applicants. Luckily, there is a growing number of colleges that offer special programs that cater to people who want to change careers and enter medicine (and already have a bachelor's degree). These post-baccalaureate programs allow older students to take pre-med courses and provide specialized counseling to aid their students in gaining admission into medical school. These programs also provide a committee letter, which is a comprehensive letter of reference that obviates an applicant's need to collect letters of recommendation from their undergraduate professors, many of whom they have not seen for years, if not decades. Special masters programs (SMPs)are also an option. For more information on post-bac and SMP programs, see "Poor GPA" in Chapter 11.

Summary

- No matter what, your life story and background are likely to have many unique aspects that can add to the culture and diversity of any student body. Identifying these special facets and writing about them honestly in your application can add depth to your application and significantly improve your chances of admission.

- Common pitfalls are when applicants mischaracterize or overemphasize their background or experiences in a self-serving way.

- Applicants invariably perform best when they can link their extracurricular activities, achievements, or leadership to a narrative that highlights their cultural or socioeconomic background or other special circumstances.

[1] https://www.aamc.org/system/files/2019-11/2019_FACTS_Table_A-14.2.pdf

[2] https://www.census.gov/quickfacts/fact/table/US/IPE120218

[3] https://www.aamc.org/system/files/reports/1/october2018anupdatedlookattheeconomicdiversityofu.s.medicalstud.pdf

[4] https://www.med.upenn.edu/admissions/entering-class-profile.html

Figure 1:
  https://www.aamc.org/system/files/2019-11/2019_FACTS_Table_A-14.1.pdf
  https://www.aamc.org/system/files/2019-11/2019_FACTS_Table_A-14.2.pdf

Figure 2:
  https://www.aamc.org/system/files/2019-11/2019_FACTS_Table_B-5.2.pdf
  https://www.census.gov/quickfacts/fact/table/US/IPE120218

Figure 3:
  https://www.aamc.org/data/facts/applicantmatriculant/157998/mcat-gpa-grid-by-selected-race-ethnicity.html

Figure 4:
  https://www.aamc.org/data/facts/applicantmatriculant/157998/mcat-gpa-grid-by-selected-race-ethnicity.html

About the Authors

Dr. Byron Lee got his B.A. from the University of California, Berkeley and M.D. degree from Harvard Medical School. He finished a medicine residency and cardiovascular fellowship at Stanford University Medical Center. He currently is Professor of Medicine in the Division of Cardiology at the University of California, San Francisco (UCSF). He has served on the admissions committee at both Harvard Medical School and UCSF.

Dr. Andrew Ko received his Sc.B. from Brown University and his M.D. degree from the Johns Hopkins School of Medicine. Following a medicine residency at the Beth Israel Hospital of Harvard Medical School, he completed a fellowship in medical oncology at Stanford University Medical Center before joining the faculty at UCSF, where he is a Professor of Medicine in the Division of Hematology/Oncology. He joined UCSF's medical school admissions committee in 2008.

Dr. Matthew Peters attended the University of California, Berkeley, where he received a degree in psychology. He was a city news reporter for his college newspaper, The Daily Californian, and later wrote news stories for a CBS affiliate in San Francisco. After graduating from UCSF School of Medicine, he started his psychiatry residency at UCSF.

Samantha An graduated with a B.S. in Business Administration from Chapman University. She is currently a freelance writer.

Made in the USA
Middletown, DE
17 October 2023